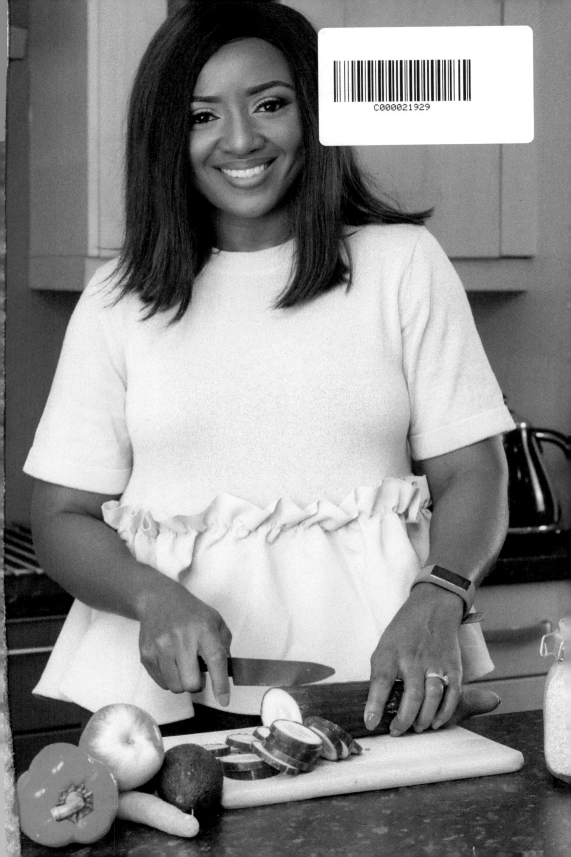

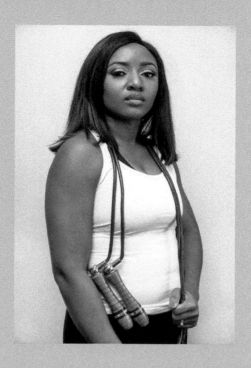

#LifestyleChangeWithApril

Your Guide to a Healthier You

April Laugh

Matador
9 Priory Business Park,
Wistow Road, Kibworth Beauchamp,
Leicestershire. LE8 0RX
Tel: 0116 279 2299
Email: books@troubador.co.uk
Web: www.troubador.co.uk/matador
Twitter: @matadorbooks

ISBN 978 1788034 647

British Library Cataloguing in Publication Data.
A catalogue record for this book is available from the British Library.

Printed and bound by CPI Group (UK) Ltd, Croydon, CR0 4YY
Typeset in 11pt Minion Pro by Troubador Publishing Ltd, Leicester, UK

Matador is an imprint of Troubador Publishing Ltd

Photography by Kareen Cox
Illustrations by Sunny Efemena
Edited by Temitayo Olofinlua

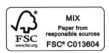

To my darling husband, who trusted me during our long-distance relationship to put him on the right path towards losing over 40kg! You are the wind beneath my wings. Thank you for your unwavering support, and for helping others to live their best life!

To my sweet mom, for laying the foundation about healthy eating. You put me in the right direction; now I can pass this on to my son, Bryan. I look forward to sharing all your yummy recipes in my next book.

Acknowledgement

Behind a fierce April Laugh are all the women on the LifestyleChangeWithApril! You are all the reason behind this book— all our hilarious conversations about weight loss, workout routines and finding a balance! You women, every single one of you— wives, mothers, career women and every thing you can possibly be—are truly amazing.

Thank you for being part of my journey, thank you for trusting me with yours. Thank you for taking good care of your bodies. Thank you for all your sweatfies and all the efforts you are making, to be a better woman! Thank you for supporting me and helping me to be better.

Here is to us, and many others to come! We do it for the 'after' pictures! Stay fierce! Stay determined! Stay sophisticated! Stay prayerful! Stay strong! Stay powerful!

To all my amazing followers on social media, thank you for cheering me on with every 'like', comment, recommendation and for believing in the April Laugh brand!

Contents

Introduction: The Road to a Healthy Lifestyle ix

Fit-ish 1
Binge Eating and How to Stop Cravings 9
Beat Bloating in a Blink 17
Drink Up. You are not Hungry 26
Rest 36
Effective Ways to Speed up Your Metabolism 47
A Practical Approach to Healthy Eating 52
Eating for a Sustained Weight Loss 67
Tips to Burn Calories and Stay Motivated 74
Weight Loss on Holiday 81
Healthy Pregnancy 90
A Simple Effective Meal Diary 103
Dear April… 121
Smash Your Fitness Goals 168

April – Detox Guide 173

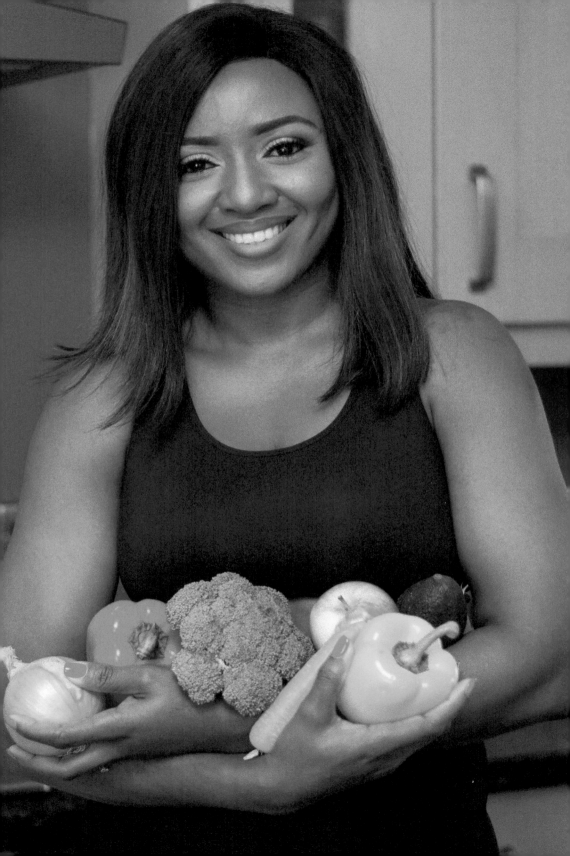

Introduction

The Road to a Healthy Lifestyle

Hello there,

My name is April. I am a certified nutritionist, fitness enthusiast, a meal plan genius, and a healthy foodie. I am passionate about helping people. Generally speaking, I am a woman trying to make a difference in the world. It is my desire for everyone that I come in contact with to live their life to the fullest!

At 30, on holiday in Miami, I was so ashamed to wear a 2-piece bikini because of the way I looked. That day, I looked at myself in the mirror and decided to live a healthier lifestyle. I had always been a size 10 but I was gradually moving to a size 12 with a huge potbelly! I was shocked by the woman I saw! That was when my journey started. Luckily, I was selected to be on a fitness challenge with TW Magazine in Lagos and I nailed it! Those twelve weeks were exciting and challenging. I went to the gym 6am daily before starting my 9-5 job. I ate clean as if my life depended on it; I prepped my meals and rarely ate junk. I also had the opportunity of working with a personal trainer and a group of amazing women I was accountable to. Boy, it paid off! I went from this flab woman to fine-ass chic wearing bodycon dresses! This drive gave me a new confidence. It gave me a bounce in my step. I was single, happy, with my abs of steel!

Then I met the man who became my husband. He was beyond fascinated at how I balanced my work schedule with my fit-life in Lagos where healthy eating is ridiculously expensive. Excitingly, I helped him lose over 40kg during our long distance relationship and he has since kept it off. This gave me the push to help other people too. Since then, I have reached out to so many women with the #LifestyleChangeWithApril 12-week fitness challenge. Seeing all these transformation pictures and reading their transformation stories, makes me the happiest woman ever!

I always feel very sad for people who starve or go on extreme fads because they want to lose weight. I know that most people desire to lose weight while they can still eat their favourite meals. I know how to make this a reality, your reality. With years of research on eating clean, and getting certified as a nutritionist, I have created meal plans that help people all over the world shed tons of pounds. All meal plans are customised to suit your desired weight loss goals and you actually EAT to lose weight. This book contains secrets to your lifestyle change.

What makes the #LifeStyleChangeWithApril different from other weight loss programmes? Your lifestyle actually changes. This comes with daily accountability, an amazing support group, fun exercise routines; these lead to a lifestyle change. I also believe in a healthy lifestyle rather than a quick diet fix. You can live your best life with April! I sincerely hope that this book will give you the need to kick-start your journey to a better you. This book is for anyone interested in living a healthier life. Weight loss may make you look good but a healthier you will feel good.

If so many people are on a bus to a place, the experience of the journey will be different for each person. Same with this lifestyle change journey. The journey is not a dash; maybe it is a marathon race in a town with many potholes along the way. As a racer, you may be tempted to give up; your enthusiasm level may drop but keep going. It is the same on the road to a lifestyle change: self-doubt may creep in; despair may walk in but mind them not, keep going. It took you so many years to get here.

The road to a lifestyle change has many bus-stops; health tips that can lead to a wholesome you, inside and out. There are tips on making the perfect meal plan for your size. There are ideas on accountability on the journey. There is information on how to get more sleep. You can learn how to lose weight on a holiday. You will know how you eat more to lose more fat, or how drinking more water is the solution to getting trapped liquid out of your system. If you are interested in increasing your metabolism, there are tricks. Some of the knowledge in this book may be strange to you, but they are tried and tested. They work.

In the last chapter of the book, women who are on the journey share their experiences; the highs and lows. We hope that these stories will inspire you to walk towards becoming a better version of you!

On your mark! Get set! Go!

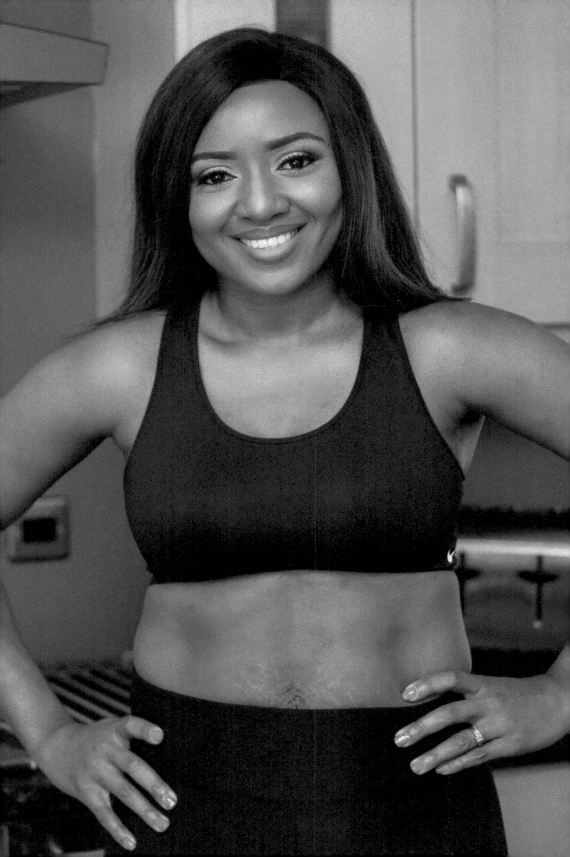

CHAPTER 1

Fit-ish

i) *(n) Semi-fit; Kinda Fit*
ii) *Someone who likes the idea of being fit but equally likes food*
iii) *(n) All the actions on the road to being fit (Nigerian language)*

Hi. My name is Joy. As my name implies, I'm a happy-go-lucky girl! I find joy, literally in everything I do. I live in Lagos with my family and I work in an investment bank. My job is pretty draining at the moment but I'm trying to find a balance with other things going on in my life. It is currently 8pm. I'm stuck in traffic. In my hand is a bottle of soft drink to keep my stomach filled. On the chair, M&S chocolates to keep my mouth busy before I get home.

With my other hand, I scroll on my Instagram feed. It is my way of keeping in touch with a world that is passing me by quickly. I move through the pictures of old school mates who are now married: "Aww, they look so in love". From one picture, I move to the next. Then stop at an old friend's pictures of her children: "These lil ones are so cute!" I comment on Adebola's Instagram pictures of her twins. Much as I try, I cannot keep up with the fast pace at which the world is moving. Whew! How can I even move when I am tied to a seat all day? That is the thought on my mind when I stumble on this page of a woman working out while she's pregnant. "Wonders shall never end! How in the world are you meant to do that? Is that even allowed? Ha! Look at her, she's even doing push-ups," I think and say out loud, even as I chuckle.

"Madam what is funny?" Fatai, my driver, asks, craning his neck to look in the front mirror, to see if everything is fine with me.

"Madam, is all well?' He asks again.

"Fatai, why not face where you are going? Do you want to drive me into the gutter tonight?"

I ignore him and continue scrolling through @fitmrsfats page on Instagram. I had to see more of this American wonder. "Na only she waka come?" Page after page, I keep loading pictures after pictures. Then, I start to see the number of women that have gone from a size 20 to size 10!

"Is this a dream?" So many "before-after" pictures that detail the transformation of different people. One woman's whose "before" goal is even my "after" goal now has abs. The more I scroll, the more pictures I see, the harder I laugh. I even saw pictures of my friend! Well, not my friend but my colleague. So, this is Folake's secret! There is a new radiance on her face these days—a bounce in her feet and her voice. She has even been parading the office with new clothes. It is just now that everything is adding up: she lost so much weight so she had to change her wardrobe. But wait a minute, Folake loves food as much as I do; her mouth is always busy. Ha! Nawa o! I would like to know how she did it though.

I don't think this woman can be of any help to me, to be honest. I have a predicament when it comes to my body. I have called it the Joy issue. Why? It seems like I am the only one in the universe who really tries to be "fitter" than she is but nothing works much. I jump rope 100 times every day. I walk around my office to count reasonable steps. I frog jump while my kettle of water is boiling yet my love handles sit smug on my waist. My arms remain fat. This is what I think my problem is: my love for food. See, I am the type who cannot let food, any type of food, from any part of the world, pass me by. My love for food is out of this world. Every time I eat a good meal, I get a foodgasm, that feeling of fulfilment, my perfect definition of heaven.

I sip from the bottle of soft drink in my hand.

Today alone, I have had two solid meals. Breakfast was ewa agonyin with fried dodo and goat meat from that woman on Victoria Island. The beans swam in oil in competition with the plantain and meat. Very sweet food. My intestines even thanked me after it with sounds of pleasure. Lunch was fairly healthy, efo riro and 1 small wrap of Amala from Mama Isale Eko. Mama Isale Eko sure knows how to cook her efo riro and make her amala so smooth that after one wrap, I am always tempted to request another. This afternoon, I refused the urge. Dinner would probably be that jollof rice from Tomi's bridal shower. Oh wait. I also had two cupcakes for snacks with my regular cappuccino decaf. This is a very good day but don't judge me abeg. I like food. I breathe food. I can't do without food. That is a fact. Even my mother knows that I was born this way and I am not complaining. Please do not complain either.

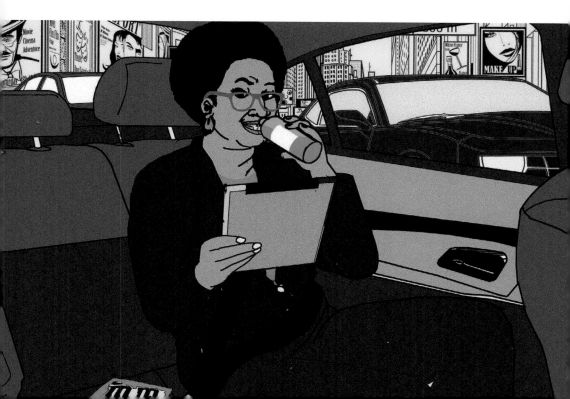

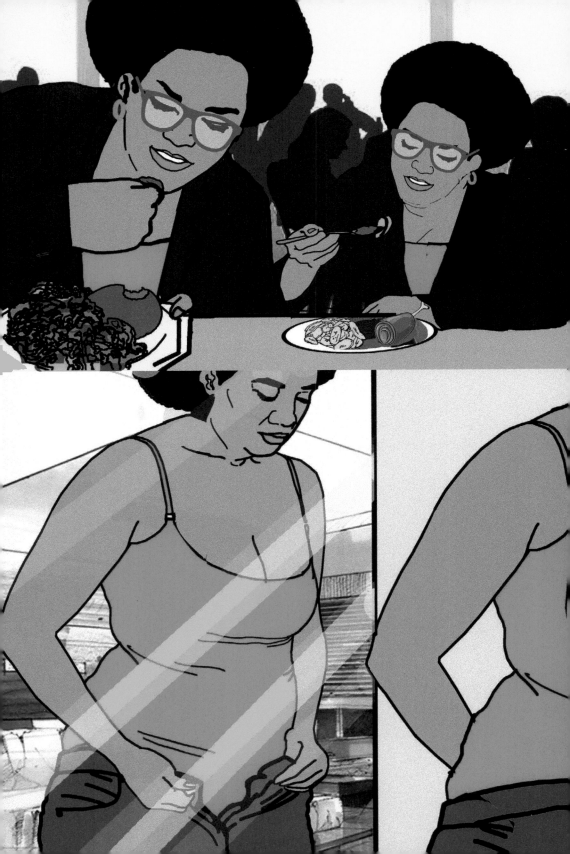

Is it your food? Is it your fat? I like my life. Just that recently, I have noticed that my clothes feel and look tighter. As much as I struggled this morning, I could not even button up my jacket. So, I let it just fly open like that. However, that moment—standing in front of the mirror struggling with my button—set the alarm off in my head. I had a conversation with two parts of me.

"Joy you are fat," one part said.

"No, I am not. I am just chubby! We all have rosy cheeks in my house," the other part of me replied.

"So why can't you button up this jacket?" The first part asked again.

"Just because I cannot button up the jacket does not mean that I am fat," the second Joy responded.

At that moment, I looked at my arms, my puffy face and I agreed: Joy you are fat. Maybe I can work on my fat arms; it is time to rock the many sleeveless dresses I am afraid to wear. Maybe my thighs as well; I have to wear that bodycon that I got as my last birthday present. My thighs even become bruised whenever I have to walk for long.

I am looking at @fitmrsfats page again. I see all these food pictures, videos and she is supposed to be helping people to lose weight? This must be jazz. How does she do it? How can I do it? Hmmm, maybe just maybe o. Maybe I should send a message to @Fitmrsfats to know how she helps people.

"Madam, we are home." Fatai says. I was so engrossed I did not realise how fast the traffic moved.

"Ha. Fatai! I wasn't even watching the road with you. We thank God. Please help me with my bags."

"Madam, you didn't finish your drink. Should I keep it for you?"

Blank stare This Fatai is one kind sha, I think but did not speak.

"Fatai, throw the drink away or you drink it!"

Prostrating with all smiles "Thank you, madam."

As I step into my house, I realise everywhere is dark. "Can someone please put on the generator?"

"Madam, I don't think…"

"You don't think what?!! Please don't tell me there's no diesel at this time! I'm going to cut off someone's head tonight! After the 5,000 naira you people collected two nights ago to fill up the tank?"

"Sorry madam. I don't think the gateman is available. Can I put it on?" Fatai asks.

"What? You are still asking?! My friend, will you keep quiet and do something! I need to workout!"

I don't even know if I should eat this jollof rice before or after I jump these ropes tonight. If I jump before I eat, won't I faint? If I jump after eating, will I vomit the food? What's the worst that can happen? Please! I'm only fat o, I didn't kill somebody! Let me eat and workout before I sleep.

Sweating profusely and gasping. I jump on the scale at the corner of the room: 75kg. Not even the smallest gram had moved.

"Mschew," I hissed loudly.

"This life a pot of beans! Hian! If this fat won't melt with all my jump ropes and Lekki Bridge running, maybe I should just contact @fitmrsfats. It's already 11pm, if I send the message now, will I be too desperate? Hmmmm, let me follow her first."

> *Dear FitMrsFats,*
>
> *I was just scrolling through Instagram tonight and stumbled on your page. What a WOW! I like what you do already and I see you like food? ☺ I'll like to be part of the AL Fithive but I have a very hectic job and I like food. I've tried to do so many things in the past few months and this is going to be my last attempt to even try to lose weight. So I hope this works for me. I can see from your profile that you're fully booked till December, does that mean I will continue to add this weight till the abroad people come in December? I can also see from your profile that you're not based in Nigeria. I hope this won't be a problem with all the Oyinbo food I see on your page? Kindly get back to me to know how this works. I am very interested.*
>
> *Thank you,*
> *Joy A.*

As I hit the send button, I quickly deleted the message! My spirit is willing to be fit but not tonight.

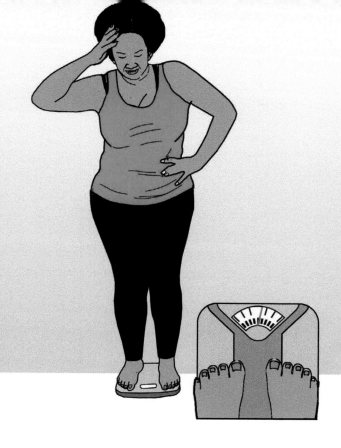

* * *

It's a beautiful morning in Lagos! The sun is shinning through my sunglasses even though it's only 7am. I'm on my way to the office, humming to "Olowogbogboro". I love driving myself to work in the morning when there is less traffic and let Fatai do the job at night. I'm going to stop at White Café for their yummy breakfast before I get to the office. I might just do a takeaway today.

Phone buzzes with a message from Instagram.

"Whatttttt! Wait. Whattttt! Didn't I delete that message from my DM last night? Is this woman a witch? She's already replied? How?! Wait sef, let me see."

Dear Joy,

Awwww. We are already friends in my head, you like food! Thank you so much for contacting me! You've come to the right place to achieve your lifestyle goals! So what exactly does the Lifestyle Change with April offer? Irrespective of the plan you're thinking of signing up for, be ready to have a change in your current eating patterns, and your exercise habits. In addition to that, you'll also be on a small, private group for personal accountability and weigh-in every two weeks.

What about exercise? We'll also provide guidance regarding an exercise regime to complement your chosen plan. The emphasis will be on a healthy, balanced diet regime which suits your activity levels. It's been amazing working with hundreds of women all over the world to achieve their set goals and I'm looking forward to working with you on your journey too. Will this be something you'd be interested in?

I look forward to reading from you.

Love, April.

CHAPTER 2

Binge Eating and How to Stop Cravings

Food for the body is not enough; there must be food for the soul
Dorothy Day[1]

Once in a while, you will find yourself over-eating or eating randomly when you are not hungry. You are out to celebrate a friend's birthday and you find yourself in the middle of a buffet. That is okay. Friends are priceless. Celebrating with friends is worth everything. What is not okay is when you order a bowl of ice-cream every night with a bucket of fried chicken because you feel some type of way! If this happens daily and you are going out of control, then you may be suffering from binge eating disorder.

According to the National Health Service (NHS)[2], a binge is an episode of excessive eating or drinking. People who binge, eat very large quantities

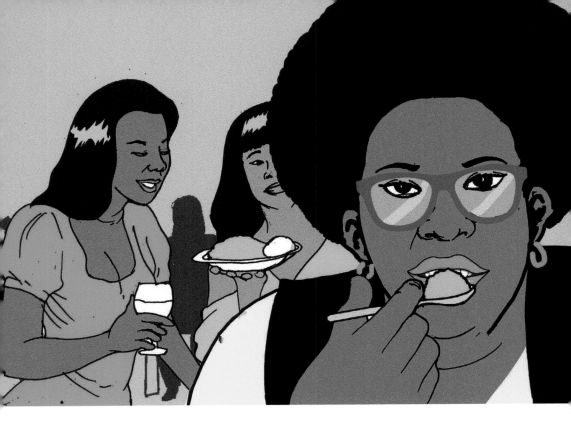

of food over a short period of time, even when they are not hungry. Signs of binge eating disorder include:

- eating much faster than normal
- eating until you feel uncomfortably full
- eating a large amount of food when you are not hungry
- eating alone or secretly because you are embarrassed about the amount of food you are consuming
- having feelings of guilt, shame or disgust after binge eating

People who regularly eat this way are likely to have a binge eating disorder. Binge eating disorder is different from eating a lot of food, from time to time. This happens, even to the best of us, when we are faced with our favourite meals. So, what makes binge eating different from eating a lot of food from time to time? Binge eaters usually feel powerless. They are unable to control themselves and stop the spoon from heading into the mouth.

"April, can I have a slice of cake since I haven't eaten anything all day? If a slice of cake is 1,500 calories and my daily limit is 1,500, can I substitute?"

Do you think a calorie is a calorie, no matter how unhealthy your meal is? No! Don't even try that! How can you compare the quality of your healthy meals to junk? Even though your body does use up the calories it needs, the quality of the food you eat will determine how fast those calories are used up and how your body uses them at the end of the day. While a bowl of brown rice will be easily digested and burned, a slice of cake will spike up your sugar levels and store up as fat few hours later.

Parties are a major source of places where your cravings come to life, especially with alcohol and small chops! However, remember that alcohol contains hundreds of calories in just one drink and of little to no nutritional value but small chops? Oh Lord! The amount of calories in those little things would ruin all your sweat for a week if not more. When you go to a party, people may pressure you to have a drink and relax, and it can be difficult to

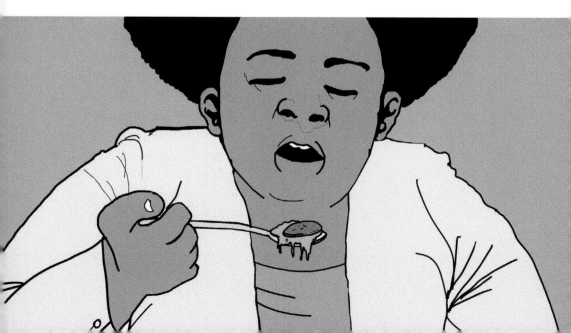

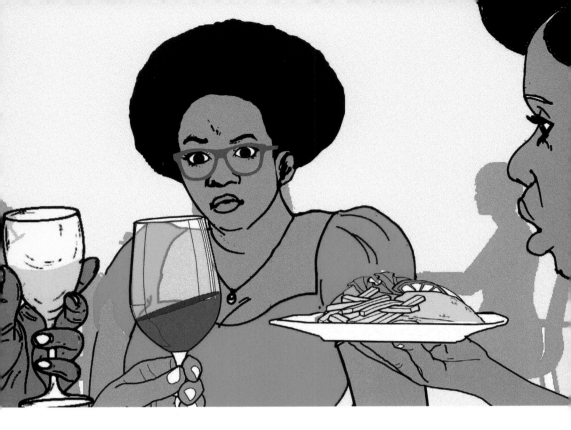

say no when they are constantly trying to convince you. The best thing is to eat before you leave home so you do not give in to party cravings.

Baby showers, weddings, birthday parties, meet-ups and other social events can also wreak havoc on your nutrition, even if you are good at resisting temptation on your own. When someone hands you a piece of cake without you asking and won't take no for an answer, it can be daunting to know what to say! *Sigh*. There are a few lies to save the day. For instance, saying that is not your favourite flavour or your stomach was upset earlier in the day will convince anyone you do not want to eat at the moment or pretending to have a chocolate allergy will get people to allow you to enjoy the party without a food hassle. For me, the most brilliant way is to joke about my new found lifestyle! (I'm on the LifestyleChangeWithApril!, join us).

You should be thinking food quality over quantity all the time! Healthy choices will get you to your goals faster while unhealthy calories slow you down. Remember, however, that while refusing foods of poor nutritional value is great, you should not stop eating good foods or start missing meals. If you do, dangerous eating habits and disorders can develop, which will give you, your friends, and your doctor a real reason to worry. Binge eating is one of such.

Some people do not even know binge eating is an illness but they go on and on complaining about not being able to stop eating! If you have been doing well on your diet, sticking to your meal plan and making daily healthy changes, then, suddenly you cannot stop thinking about popcorn or small chops or ice-cream or a burger. Is it hunger, or is it a craving? Sadly, many of us have lost the ability to tell the difference between the two. Hunger is the body's way of telling you it needs more food. If you crave fat, salt, or sugar, you can bet you are not feeling true hunger. Why are you not craving an apple? *side eye* Cravings are your body's way of telling you what it wants or needs. Once you get to the root cause of your cravings, you can take steps to send them out of the window.

Most cravings stem from feelings of deprivation, poor blood sugar control, or an unmet emotional need. There are some cravings that are stimulated by the flavour-enhancing chemicals in processed and junk foods. Some individuals, especially those with insulin resistance or type 2 diabetes, have cravings for carbohydrates that seem to get stronger as more carbs are consumed. This is due to rapidly rising and falling glucose levels.

You may eat to the point of discomfort, and then be plagued by feelings of guilt, shame, or depression afterwards. You may beat yourself up for your lack of self-control, or worry about what compulsive eating will do to your body. As powerless as you may feel about your eating disorder, it is important to know that binge eating disorder is treatable. Yes, you can learn to break the binge eating cycle, develop a healthier relationship with food, and feel good about yourself again. But first, it is important to find the cause of your binge eating. Once you discover the root cause of your cravings, you are on your road to stopping it. Here are some tips to guide you on that journey:

Eat Enough, often Enough

Can't stop thinking about food? The question is what kind of food are you craving? There are chances that you might actually be hungry. If you find yourself craving foods that are typically considered healthy, such as meats, fruits, or vegetables, give in to your cravings. Your body is telling you it needs more nutrients. To keep cravings away, eat a small, healthy meal, approximately 200 calories, six times, a day.

Avoid Artificial Sweeteners

Aspartame, sucralose, and MSGs enhance the flavour of our foods. Unfortunately, these chemicals have also been shown to create a hunger response in some individuals, even after they have eaten. Stop your cravings by reducing the amount of chemically-enhanced, processed food you eat. Prepare your own foods; this empowers you to know what goes into your food and into your body. Eat a small amount of real sugar on occasion instead of large amounts of artificial sweeteners every day.

Carbs Create Cravings

If you are diabetic, pre-diabetic, or insulin-resistant, you probably know what it is like to daydream about carbohydrates. It is because your body does not use glucose correctly, so it constantly craves sugar – and other carb-rich foods – causing a jump in blood glucose levels. Choose foods that are low in carbohydrates, or whole grain foods with plenty of fibre. These foods do not stimulate cravings the way processed flour products do.

Discover What You are Really Hungry For

If you find that you are hungry most of the time, you should take a moment to sit down and reflect on what you are hungry for. Food has a strong emotional connection for many of us, and it can be difficult to discern real hunger from boredom or loneliness or even depression. Sometimes food is just an easy accessible option to quell a desire for something else. You may actually not be hungry for food. If you are bored, you may feel better when you are in contact with friends. If you are lonely, you may just be hungry for a call with your Mum. If you are depressed, you may just need to speak with your psychiatrist. Sometimes a hug or a new activity can satisfy our needs much more than extra food can. Food is not the answer to all hunger. Find what you are hungry for.

Evaluate Your Diet

If your cravings persist after taking the above steps, your diet might not be providing all the nutrition you need. Start a food diary and write down all the foods you eat for a week or two, and then have a nutritionist evaluate your diet. They can recommend dietary changes or find substitutions that will reduce your cravings.

Eat What You Want (In Moderation)

Of course, everyone gets stuck in a food rut every now and then. Your cravings could be a signal that you are bored with your eating plan and need a little something to boost your morale. If that is the case, go ahead and eat what you crave, but keep it in moderation. Instead of having a box of pizza, have a slice and give the rest to your neighbours. Have a cupcake, but increase your exercise to compensate for the extra calories. You feel like eating something sweet? Why not pack on so much fruits loaded with nutrients instead of empty sugars. Almost any food can be an occasional part of a healthy diet.

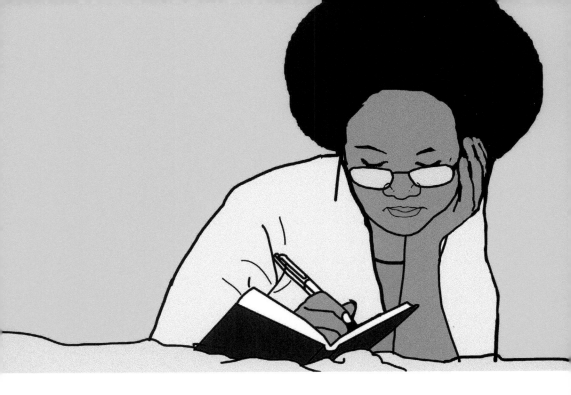

Cravings are your body's way of telling you what it wants or needs. Once you get to the root cause of your cravings, you can take steps to send them packing – permanently.

Chapter 3
Beat Bloating in a Blink

OMG! You're pregnant! No ma. I'm just bloated!

"Hey Fithive! It's time for another progress picture! So far, you've spent 8 weeks on the LifestyleChangeWithApril and I expect to see your abs by now! Please send all progress pictures in by 9am tomorrow morning.

P.S This is an AL Fithive broadcast, you don't have to reply. Thank you!"

9a.m. Fisayo has just sent in her progress pictures to April.

"Yay!"

"This my coach! Always flattering someone. Abeg, I'm buying a new mirror tomorrow."

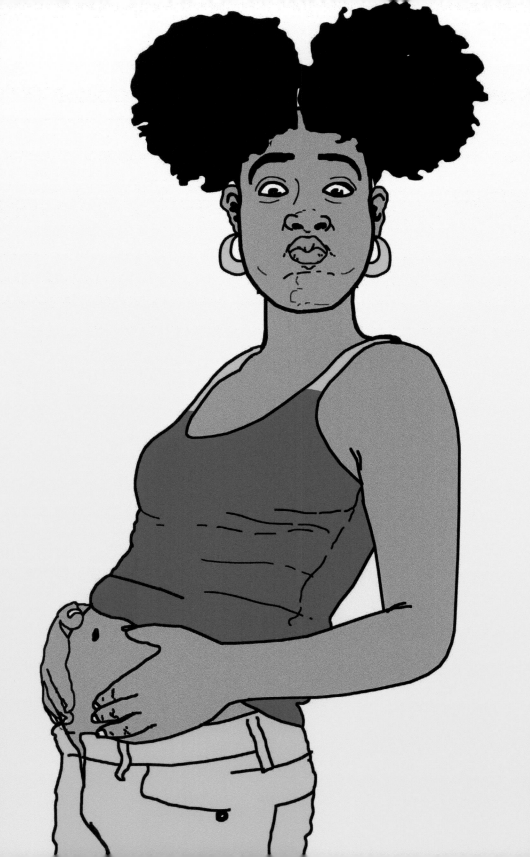

"You're pregnant!!! You didn't tell me!"

"No, ma. I'm just bloated. April, I'm always bloated please. I can't seem to drink enough water or eat enough veggies to feel better. Sometimes, it can be very painful."

You have been eating right and exercising, doing all the things April asked you to do in order to lose fat and get healthy. You have been putting into practice the words of this book from the first page but when you step on the scale, you get a nasty shock: you have gained five pounds! What did you do wrong? Absolutely nothing! Everyone experiences unexpected weight gain from time to time. This can be caused by water retention, also known as bloating. Bloating can be very discouraging to dieters, but it is important to remember that the weight gain is temporary. You can lose the water weight as fast as you gained it by following these simple rules:

1. Reduce your carb intake

Carbohydrates give us quick energy, but they also make us retain water. When stored in the body, carbohydrates attract water. The end result is a puffier appearance, tighter clothes, and a few extra pounds on the scale. To reduce bloating, eat fewer carbs. Note that this does not mean you need to eliminate all carbohydrates. Simply avoid sugar, starch, and any product made from refined white flour. Instead, eat protein, healthy fats, vegetables, and products made from ground flax seed. You will see a visible reduction in your bloating after one to two days. The strategy is simple: eat fewer carbs and exercise more. Do a mixture of cardio exercise and strength training, and eat only protein and healthy carbohydrates, like fruits and vegetables, to fuel your workouts.

2. Again, drink more water

Quick: make a fist. Do your hands feel tight and puffy? If you wear rings, do they leave deep impressions in your skin after you remove them? These are

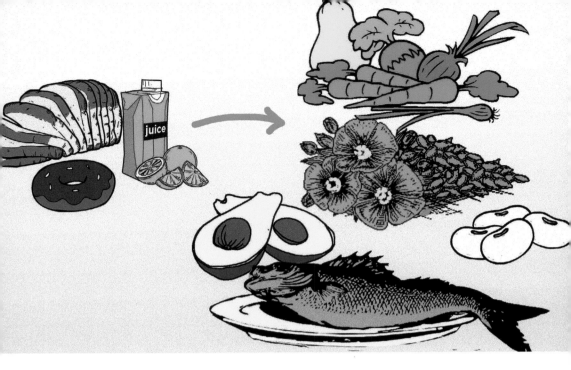

sure signs of bloating, probably stemming from dehydration. Water is a sure cure for this type of bloating.

When your body does not have enough water, it starts to hold on to every bit of fluid it has access to. This causes the fluid to build up inside you, leaving you bloated and sluggish. To overcome this survival mechanism, you will need to drink a lot of water. How much is a lot? At least 64 oz over the course of a few hours. Another sure sign of dehydration is yellow urine, no it is not fever, your body just needs more water. You can tell your dehydration is being corrected when you start to pass clear urine.

3. Cut out the extra salt

Sodium is a necessary mineral, but a diet heavy in processed and fast foods provides far more sodium than necessary. Unnecessary sodium is not healthy. The human body requires only 500mg of sodium daily, but many of us routinely take in 6,000mg or more each day! All of this extra salt can have a detrimental effect on your health and your waistline. Sodium acts as an irritant to your muscles and organs. In order to dilute this effect, your body will retain water. This is why excess salt consumption leads to bloating in so many people. To avoid this, eat as many whole, unprocessed foods as possible. Use potassium chloride as a salt substitute, and drink plenty of water to flush your system.

4. Caffeine: A quick and "dirty" trick

Caffeine has both laxative and diuretic effects. Simply put, it makes you pass waste materials and fluids at a faster rate. If you need to look your best for a special event, but yet to lose the bloat, drink some coffee along with 8 glasses of water. This should get things moving!

Remember that caffeine is simply a quick fix, and should not be used as a long-term weight loss strategy. This method will result in a loss of temporary water weight only. Go back to your healthy diet plan as soon as possible, and follow the preceding tips to keep bloating at bay. Bloating can make you look and feel bad, but these tricks will help you fit into your skinny jeans in no time!

Five Secrets to Getting a Flat Belly

As dieters, we all dream of having tight, toned stomachs with sexy six-packs. Unfortunately, abdominal fat is not only dangerous, it is just plain hard to get rid of. For many of us, the midsection seems to be the first place we pack on extra pounds, and the last place we lose them. They may be difficult but not impossible to lose. So, do not give up yet! Here are five proven secrets you can use to get a flatter stomach while you work to reduce that stubborn belly fat.

Secret #1: Reduce overall body fat

There is no such thing as spot reduction. That is, you can't lose fat in your stomach area without losing fat everywhere else. To get the lean stomach you want, you need to reduce your overall body fat percentage. This can only be done through a healthy diet and exercise regimen that combines aerobic exercise with strength-training.

Start today by researching a food plan and exercise routine you will enjoy. The most successful plans feature diets high in lean protein and complex carbohydrates, plus cardio exercise and strength-training three to five times a week.

Secret #2: Fill up on fibre and protein

Snacking on the wrong foods can sabotage your tummy-busting efforts. Keep your hunger—and your waistline—in check by filling up on whole grain oatmeal, fruits and vegetables, beans, lean meats, nuts, and olives. Foods that are high in Omega-3 fatty acids, such as fish, help counteract the fattening stress hormone: cortisol. Cortisol sends signals to the body that cause it to go into survival mode, storing fat all over, but particularly around the midsection. Reduce your cortisol levels, and your body will start to burn through those fat stores again. You can reduce cortisol today by relaxing and eating foods high in Omega-3s.

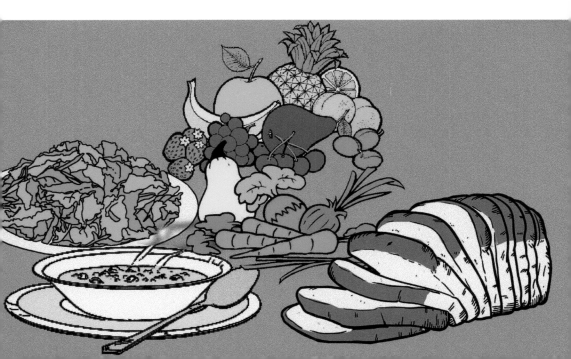

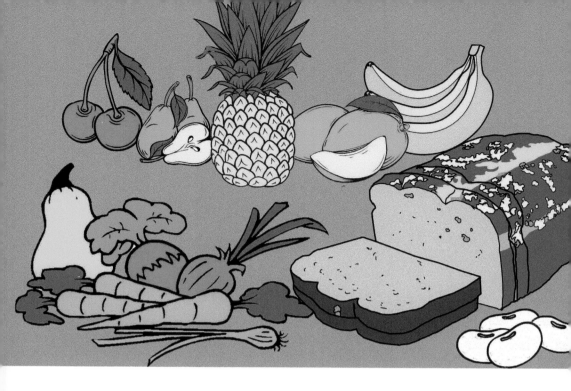

Secret #3: Stay away from salt and sugar

Carbohydrates cause us to retain water, hence the "hydrates" suffix. This can result in bloating, especially in the tummy area. Salt is another notorious bloat-inducer. Instead of loading up on table salt, try smaller amounts of sea salt, or a salt substitute. For quick stomach shrinkage, reduce the number of carbs you consume each day. The ones you do eat should come from whole grains, nuts, fruits and vegetables. These complex carbohydrates help regulate hunger and minimize cravings.

Secret #4: Strengthen your core with regular sculpting exercises

Exercise will help remove the layer of fat that hides your abs from view. It will also help shape those hidden muscles so that they will look great when they finally make their appearance. A strong core will also help you stand and sit upright, which has a two-fold benefit: good posture makes you look slimmer, and also gives you ample opportunities to work those abs by holding them taut

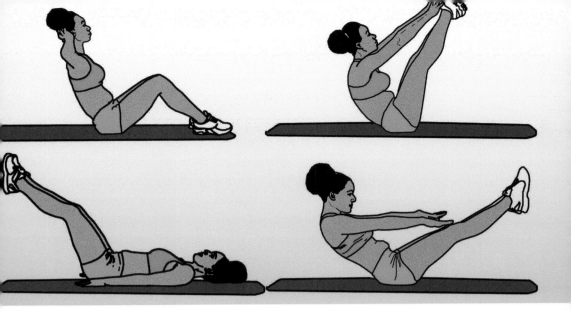

as you walk or sit. For the strongest, most sculpted abs, do core-strengthening exercises like sit-ups, V-ups, leg lifts, or Pilates three or more times a week.

Secret #5: Drink water to flush fat away

It might seem counter-intuitive to load up on water when you already feel bloated, but the fluid you consume actually helps your body get rid of the fluid it is holding on to. Bloating occurs when the body is dehydrated. In an

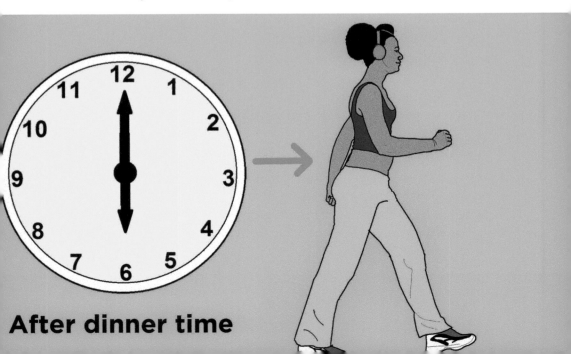

After dinner time

effort to preserve its vital fluids, the body holds onto every bit of water it has, resulting in puffiness in the hands and abdomen. The only way to counteract this is to drink enough water to make your body feel safe again, allowing it to flush the retained fluid from its system.

A flat stomach is something you must earn over time, but that does not mean you cannot make some quick fixes today!

Stand up tall! You are already making progress toward your goal.

Chapter 4

Drink Up. You are not Hungry

"How many glasses of water have you had today?"

:s

"I'm really struggling with that. I think I had three glasses. Not sure, do you want me to drink more?"

:S

"Yes! You are not hungry, you are thirsty! Drink up!"

"Wait, does my coffee count? The green tea? Please, I'm asking for a friend. Please say yes."

Shaking my head.

Okay, let us speak about this water drinking issue. Why do people find it hard to drink water? We are often told to drink up and stay hydrated but do you know why it is so important? Water can contribute to weight loss–even fast weight loss—in several ways. Yes ma'am, if you are trying to lose weight, you need h20! The "water solution" may be the missing puzzle in your weight loss hustle!

First, since our bodies need water to survive, they have a self-defence reaction when we do not consume enough water. In response to dehydration, they start to hold on to every bit of fluid they get. This is called fluid retention, or bloating, and it can cause the scale to leap up by several pounds.

The cure for bloating is easy: drink more water. If you drink at least eight glasses a day which is approximately three litres a day, your body will start to let go of the fluid it has been retaining. Your waist will shrink unbelievably, and you will lose some superfluous pounds. Water can be really helpful for weight loss. It is 100 per cent calorie-free; helps you burn

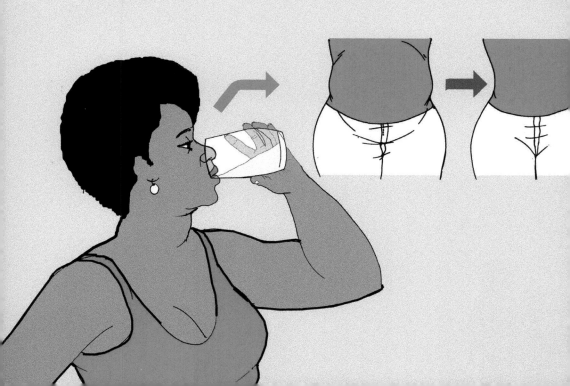

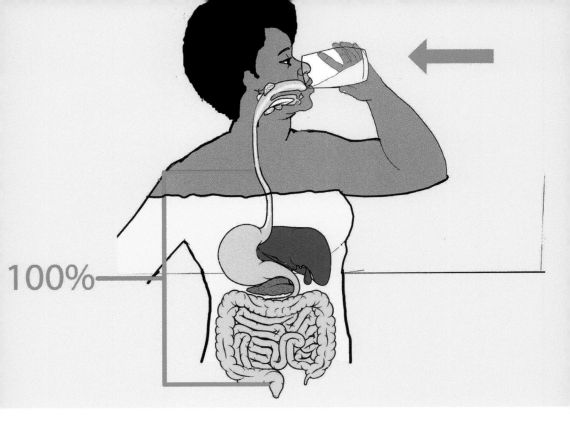

100%

more calories and may even suppress your appetite if consumed before meals.

How do you tell if you are bloated? Clench your hands into fists. Do they feel tight and puffy? Are your rings leaving indentations on your fingers? If so, you might be bloated, and water can help right away. Go on. Take a glass of water. Take some more.

Secondly, water acts as a vitamin delivery system. The vitamins you consume through food and supplements are distributed throughout your body if you are properly hydrated. If you have not had enough fluids, the vitamins will have trouble getting where they need to go.

Water is even good for skin. One way to know whether you are taking enough water is to look at your skin. If it is shining, you may be getting enough water. If it is wrinkly, you may not be getting enough water and need to increase water intake. Different seasons of the year also affect the amount of water intake; during the dry season, you may get dehydrated often, so drink more water. However, dry or rainy season; winter or summer, drink water every time.

Finally, water keeps our organs functioning at their highest level. This directly affects your body's ability to burn fat on the long run. This explains why you feel like drinking a gallon during or after your workouts.

You see, our bodies have a natural filtration system that gets rid of toxins and built-up fluid: the kidneys. But the kidneys need plenty of water to do their job properly. If you do not drink enough water, the kidneys have to call on the liver for back-up filtration. While the liver is busy helping out the kidneys, it is not metabolising fat as efficiently as it should, and more of the food you eat will be stored as fat.

You can avoid this situation by drinking at least 64 ounces of pure drinking water each day. That is eight cups of water daily. A more customised approach is to drink 1 ounce of water for every 2 pounds of body weight. Thus, a 150 pound woman would need eight glasses of water each day. If you do a lot of sweating, or if you have a medical condition that leaves you chronically dehydrated (like diabetes) you will need extra hydration.

There are so many easy ways to maximise drinking water daily. Let me share some with you six tips that keep me gulping. Many of them I have tried because the struggle to increase water intake is real.

1. Set a Specific Goal for the Day

Maybe you already drink a fairly decent amount of water every day; clap for yourself. Then, drink some more. Maybe you hardly drink any. Start by figuring out how much you consume now, and how much you should consume. One of the easy ways to set water-drinking goals is by setting "small" goals, like water to drink for a day. Then zero in on real numbers: like going from four to nine glasses per day. This is also a fun challenge you can run with a friend. Do not worry, you cannot choke on water. You may just visit the toilet some more. Not bad. Your body is functioning, and water is helping it to run.

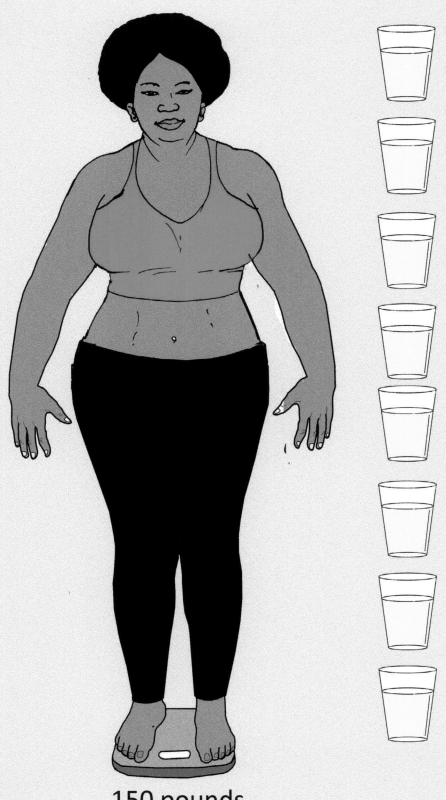

150 pounds

2. Invest in a Water Bottle

It is not only children who need water bottles, adults also do. With a water bottle, you are sure that you have water at your "finger tips" literally. Then, use it. Your water bottle should be used for what it is meant—carrying water around. Do not dump it in the fridge. Then actually drink the water. Pick a colour that you find attractive. For me, the fancier the bottle, the more I drink. The more you drink, the happier your body, the more your skin will thank you.

3. Drink from a Bottle.

I know this might sound manner-less but—before you judge me—it works for me. I reckon it is a way of tricking my body—or is it my brain now?—to drink more water. Maybe it is the fun of gulping that makes me take more, I do not know but bottle on the lips, several gulps down my throat, I realise the bottle is almost empty. Then, I psych myself up to finish the bottle. Then, repeat the act before I feel thirsty again; note, before the thirst. Once you are thirsty, your body is already in need of water. Do not wait for your body to ask you; satisfy the thirst before it even begins. Your body will thank you.

4. Add a Favourite Flavour for Variety

You think water has a bland taste? Wait till you meet water flavoured with berries, citrus, or lavender. Any fruit flavour can add taste to the water. The flavour not only gets you to drink the water but the nutrients will also go into your body. It is just like using one stone to kill two birds. You can find these and other ideas for infused water on aprillaugh.co.uk.

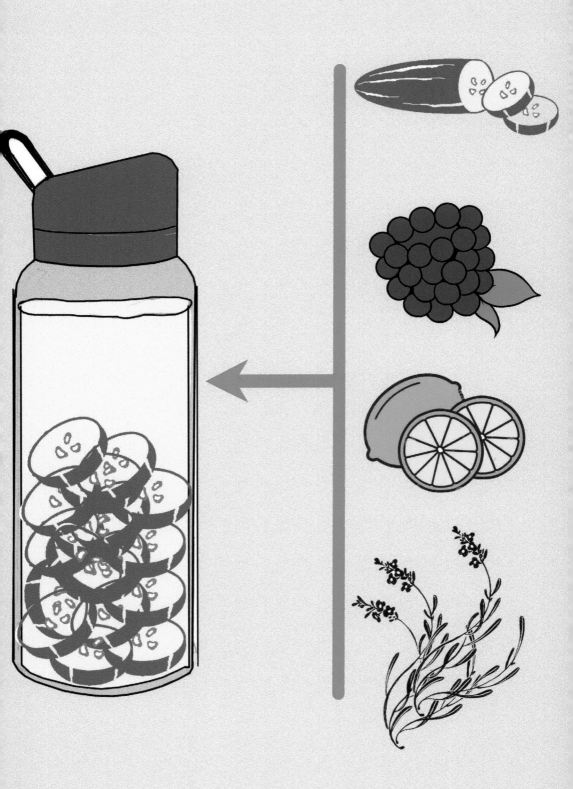

5. Compete

Wrangle up friends, co-workers or your children to join you. For example, make it a goal to drink at least five glasses during the workday; then set up shared calendar reminders to make sure you are all on track. Feeling extra competitive? Place a friendly bet.

6. Hydrate with Water-based Foods

Watermelons in all its red and sweet glory, anyone? There are also vegetables with high water content. This includes cucumber and lettuce, consisting of 96 per cent water. Zucchini, radish and celery are 95 per cent water. Ninety-four per cent of tomato's weight is water, and green cabbage is 93 per cent water. Other vegetables that contain water include cauliflower, eggplant, red cabbage, peppers, broccoli and spinach. Water-based foods guarantee

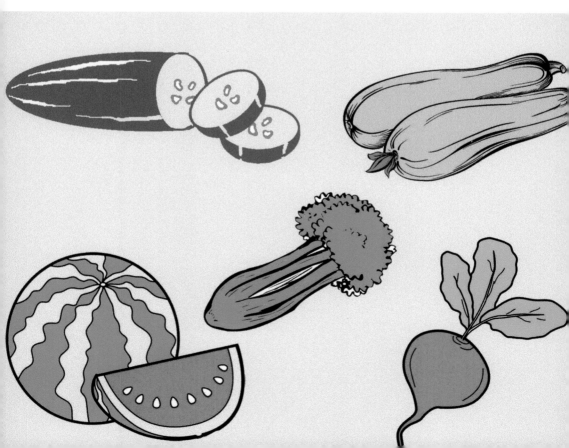

a great way to pack on vitamins that your body needs and get all the water as well.

A Drinking Regimen

Do not roll your eyes. You see when you notice that you are not getting enough water; you have to be deliberate on this journey. The water will not evaporate from the atmosphere into your body; it must come through your mouth. Guzzle a full glass during the parts of your day where you already have a routine—like when you wake up, after breakfast, before lunch, and before dinner. Adding a drink to existing regimens will make you more likely to a) remember it, and b) actually do it. So, it is nothing complicated, your water regimen likely would look something like this:

- When you wake up: 2 Glasses
- After Breakfast: 1 Glass
- Midday: 1 Glass
- Before Lunch: 1 Glass
- Lunch: 1 Glass
- After lunch: 1 Glass
- Before Dinner: 1 Glass
- Dinner: 1 Glass
- Anytime you forget: double the glass of water ☺

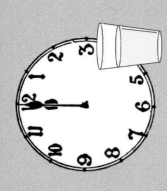
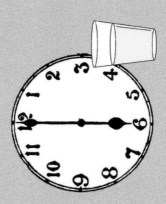
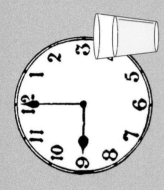
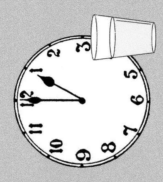
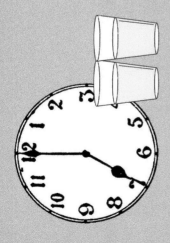
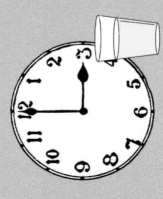
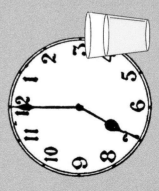

Chapter 5

Rest

*"Almost everything will work again if you unplug it for a few minutes…
including you!"*

Anne Lamott[6]

"April. I'm tired of this journey. I'm really exhausted and it's so frustrating. I have tried a lot of things but I end up getting even more frustrated. My work is consuming. My baby is demanding. My hubby doesn't seem to understand my frustrations. I try to eat clean and burn those calories but I'm feeling burnt out. Have you ever signed up someone like me? I just want to take a break and start when things are a bit settled in my life. Sorry, good morning."

"Awwwww, good morning Jay! There's no point asking how you are with this. Sorry mama! I totally understand where you're coming from and I can only wish that things are a bit better for you at home and at work. However, quitting is not an option around here. You have to keep pushing through and keep making everyday happen. Do you know what's going to happen when you take a break?

1.   You don't care
2.   The journey remains stagnant
3.   You give up
4.   You eat rubbish
5.   You pile up unwanted pounds!

What's the worst that can happen if you keep pushing? Please tell me, how many hours of sleep do you get daily? "

"April, with all these problems, sleeping is not important o! I barely get five hours daily. On great weekends when hubby is home to take care of the kids, I do six hours. Is that any good?

:o   Oh no! You need to REST!

CLOSE YOUR EYES AND REST

When you think of weight-loss measures, sleep is not usually the first activity that comes to mind. Yet, sleep is one of the most important things you can do when you are trying to lose weight.

Just like staying hydrated, adequate sleep benefits the dieter in many ways. First and foremost, sleep relieves stress. Stress is actually counterproductive to weight loss. That is because stress triggers a chemical reaction in our bodies that actually promotes weight gain.

Think about our ancestors. They stored body fat to help them survive through times of famine. Therefore, whenever their bodies were stressed—as in times of starvation—a hormone called cortisol was released. Cortisol tells our bodies to save up their fat stores in preparation for hard times ahead.

Today, we have more stress than ever before due to job schedules, family obligations, overcrowding, and financial concerns. We are bombarded with information and advertisements. Many of us work around the clock to make ends meet. Add to that many of us who have sedentary jobs that keep us on

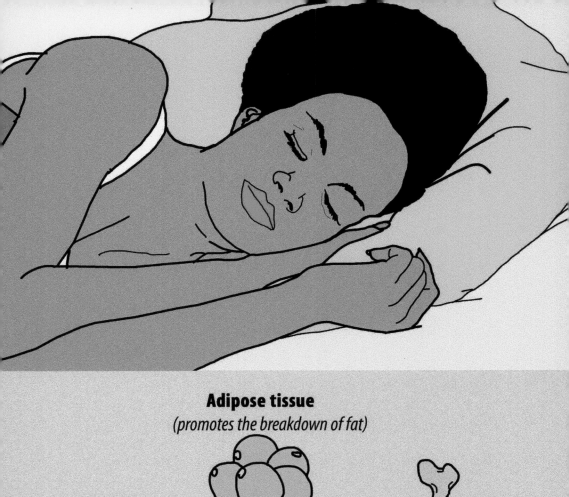

Adipose tissue
(promotes the breakdown of fat)

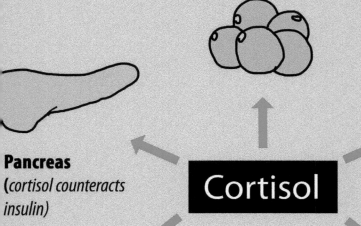

Bone
(reduces bone formation)

Pancreas
(cortisol counteracts insulin)

Cortisol

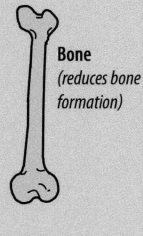

Muscle
(decreasing amino acid uptake by muscle)

Liver
(glucose genration)

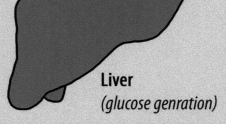

the same spot for hours. Add to that the kind of meals that we eat—packed with preservatives. Add to that a cycle of self-imposed famine in the form of dieting, and it is no wonder people are more stressed out–and fatter–than ever.

Sleep soothes the mind and body, gives us a chance to slow down and process the events of our day. Sleep speaks to the body; it tells it to replace cortisol production with endorphin production. Endorphins are feel-good chemicals that relieve stress and give us a general sense of well-being. You wake up feeling better and brighter, endorphins have oiled the wheels of your body, washed every part of it clean, making the body feel generally new.

Finally, sleep gives our bodies the opportunity to repair themselves. If you exercise, and especially if you do strength-training, you might end up with achy muscles because exercise and weight-lifting cause microscopic tears throughout your muscle tissue. When you sleep, these tears are repaired, rebuilding your muscle tissues stronger than before. This leaves you with more lean muscle mass, which means you burn more calories all day and all night, even when you sleep.

In spite of its many benefits, adequate sleep is something few of us enjoy. Studies have shown that most people do not get the 7 to 10 hours of sleep that their bodies require. Insufficient sleep can have a direct impact on how much weight you lose or gain. In need of sleep badly, let us help you with these few tips:

1. How much sleep do you get?

Before you even start sleeping, let us see how much sleep you get in order to determine how much more you need to get. Look at the amount of sleep you get each night. You do not need a calculator to do this. ☺ When did you sleep last night? When did you get up this morning? Any naps during the day? Is it enough? We all have the same number of hours in a day and we have to carve out more hours of sleep from these same 24 hours. Let us learn how in number 2.

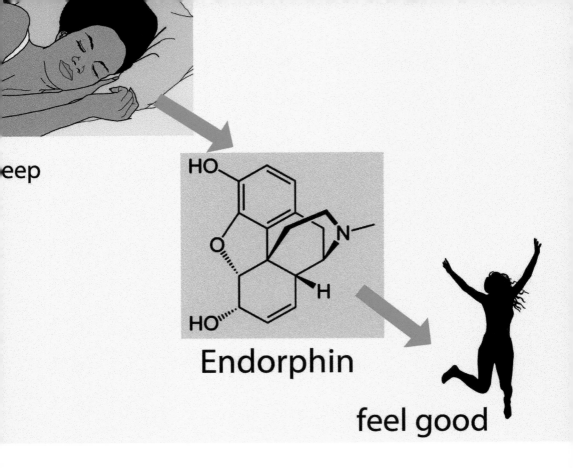

eep

Endorphin

feel good

2. Cut out the sleep deprivers

Ask yourself: what is keeping you from sleeping more? These are the sleep deprivers. Sometimes the answer is obvious, like a demanding work schedule or a new born baby—not much that many can do with this, except one has help; or a demanding work schedule. Other common culprits include too much computer time before bed—computer and video games stimulate the brain, preventing it from winding down in preparation for sleep; alcohol consumption; and insomnia due to stress or anxiety. So, what can you do? Cut them out. Avoid drinking caffeine after noon.

Had a tiring day at work? You do not need these deprivers—some are actually (addictive) habits—before you hit the bed. You know what happens many times: let me quickly check my Facebook status; let me quickly keep up with what is happening on Twitter, I will take only five

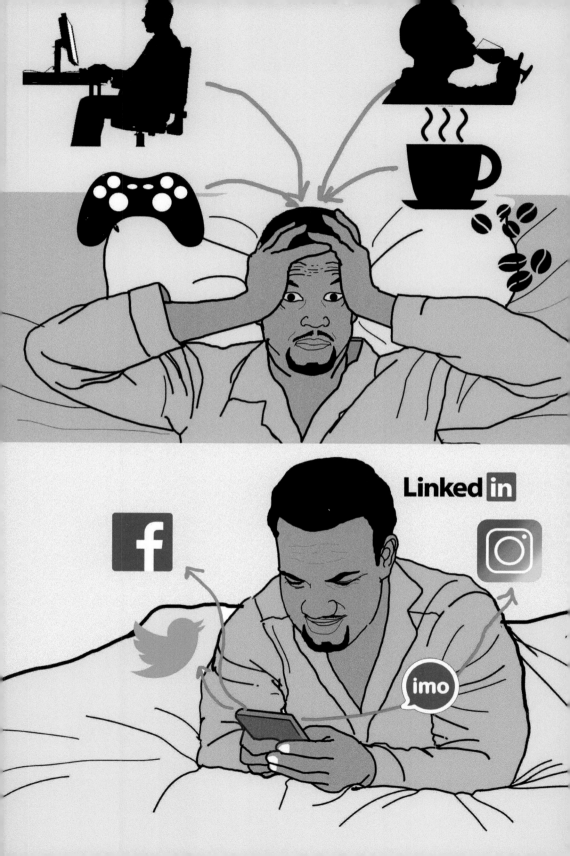

minutes then switch off. Then, five minutes becomes thirty, and then one hour, and then Twitter leads to several pages of tabs on your phone. You know what: do not start this after a busy day. Get home; get a good meal and unplug, not plug in. Oh you are not sleeping, actually shut your eyes and fix your mind on something beautiful, soon, you will be lost in lalaland and it is a new day. Your body will be filled with good vibes that make your eyes see clearer and you will be ready to take on the day with new vigour.

3. Shut your (worrying!) mind

Have you ever been sleeping and your mind seems to be awake? It is running through how your day went or your to-do list for the next day. Or it is making plans for the owambe on Saturday? Or it is taking you through the list of worries: unpaid school fees and rent? Or it is taking you through Nigeria's many troubles: you have not had light in months; you will head into the crazy traffic in the morning or the politicians who refuse to be accountable? The list is endless. Pause. Just hold it. The act of worrying, especially before

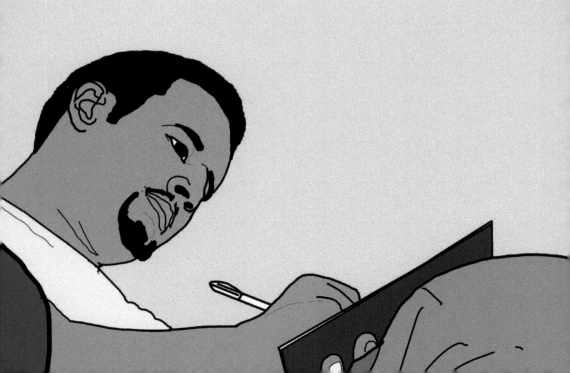

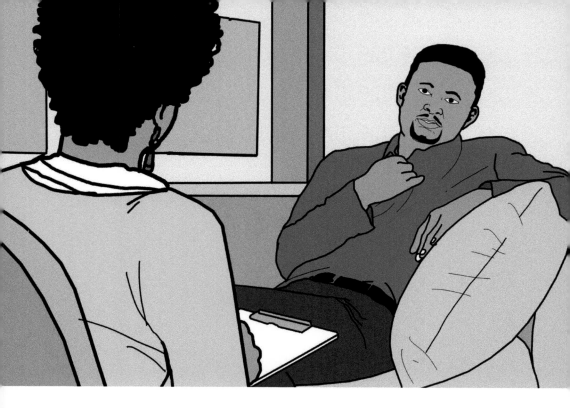

sleep, is just like a buzzing mosquito in your ears that you cannot kill. It does not allow you to sleep and if you leave it there, it will bite you and maybe give you malaria. In this case, it will stimulate hormones that will keep the calories growing. Then, wear and tear sets in. The items on your worrying list remain and you are not better for it.

So what can you do? Write. You want to remember what happens during your day? Get a journal. You may even want to create one online. Once done, shut down. And sleep. You want to figure out the things you want to do tomorrow? Write it on your to-do list, or even type it on your phone. What does this do for you? You have shifted everything from your worrying mind. And the next day, you can pick up your to-do list and start ticking off the items once they are done. The sheer joy that comes with that cannot be compared with anything. And yes, hypertension, high blood pressure and all the other issues that come with worrying about things you cannot control are far from you. And yes, the fat too :)

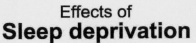

Effects of
Sleep deprivation

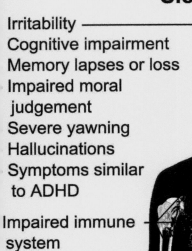

Irritability
Cognitive impairment
Memory lapses or loss
Impaired moral
    judgement
Severe yawning
Hallucinations
Symptoms similar
    to ADHD

Impaired immune
system

Risk of diabetes
Type 2

- Increased heart rate variability
- Risk of heart disease

- Increased
    reaction time
- Decreased accuracy
- Tremors
- Aches

Other:
- Growth suppression
- Risk of obesity
- Decreased
    temperature

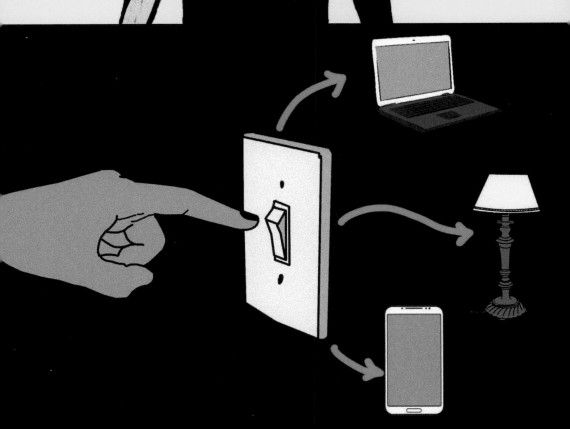

4. Manage your stress levels

Do what you can to manage your stress level while you are awake. Get some exercise each day, in the sunlight if possible. Actions in number three will also help your manage your stress levels. The journaling does not work for you? You may consider speaking to a trusted friend or an advisor; sometimes, speaking about it, especially with someone ready to listen, or someone who can help you think through the issue, helps. Yoga and meditation can also help. Never use sleep aids unless your doctor gives you the go-ahead, as they can become addictive.

5. Get Ready to Sleep:

First, be ready to sleep whenever sleep beckons. The body has a way of demanding what it needs—especially sleep—when it wants. You either pay now—by actually sleeping—or pay later, with direr consequences. So, make

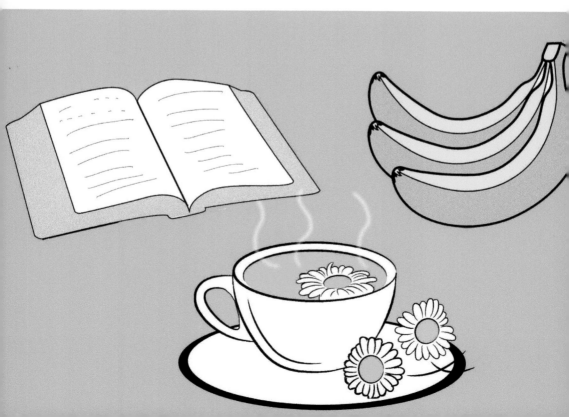

it a practice to take power naps when you can. It is an effective way to get more sleep. When last did you "see Esther"—sorry have a siesta?

Second, make sure your bedroom is conducive to a good night's sleep. If noises tend to wake you during the night, invest in a cheap pair of foam earplugs, or drown out background noise with a fan. Make sure the room is dark, and turn off any electronic devices that have flashing lights. Wind down before bed with a warm bath, a cup of chamomile tea, and a book. You can also eat a banana before bed to help you get restful sleep throughout the night.

See you in the morning!

Chapter 6

Effective Ways to Speed up Your Metabolism

April, is there anything I can do to speed up my metabolism? I attend kickboxing classes 3 times a week, I run 10km every other morning but this weight won't shift! I've tried all sorts of detox, I'm the queen of yo-yo dieting but isn't working out enough to make things change? You're the my last resort to lose this weight otherwise, I'll be going for a gastric bypass.

"Gas-kini! Calm down ma. It's not this serious. Remember you're in your 40s and while it takes longer for you to burn those calories, your body has also been used to a certain way of eating and this lifestyle change requires a lot of patience."

We all have that one friend that eats like an elephant but does not get fat. We all have that sibling that eats a mountain of food but with a stomach like a slate, even right after eating. "Where does all the food go? You eat all the food but we do not see it on your body," we joke some times. It is all in the metabolism, different bodies, different metabolism. Do not hate. Just find out what suits your body!

First let us talk about the different things we do not know about metabolism. Did you know that different diets are the main causes of slow metabolism? It is sad but true: the more diets you go on, the more damaged and inefficient your metabolism becomes. If you have been a chronic yo-yo dieter for years, you might feel like your metabolism is broken beyond repair. Some life-long dieters find that they gain weight when they eat anything approaching a healthy number of calories each day. That is a demoralising problem, but do not give up just yet! There is a fast and easy way to get your metabolism back up to speed.

The only way to a faster metabolism is *more food*

Do not scream yet. Lol! I honestly do not know why you are so scared of eating. So how does one speed up their metabolism after years of ravaging diets? As stated above, more food is the key. You need to nourish your body to encourage it to heal. This might sound too good to be true. After all, if all it takes to lose weight is to eat more food, why doesn't everyone do it? It is not as easy as it sounds. When you start to eat normally again, you will almost certainly gain weight. This quick gain scares many dieters, sending them back to the near-starvation diets they were accustomed to. Yet, if you wait it out, the scale will start to move in the right direction once more. Remember, it took your body a while to reset its metabolic rate to a slower speed. It will take just as long, if not longer, for it to speed back up.

There are some things you can do to minimise the waiting period. First, calculate how many calories you would need with a healthy BMR (Basal Metabolic Rate). Start eating that number of calories each day. It might feel like a lot of food at first, but just remember that your body is repairing itself, so it needs plenty of fuel.

> *Your BMR (Basal Metabolic Rate) is an estimate of how many calories you'd burn if you were to do nothing but rest for 24 hours. It represents the minimum amount of energy needed to keep your body functioning, including breathing and keeping your heart beating.*
>
> *Your BMR does not include the calories you burn from normal daily activities or exercise.*
>
> $$\text{BMR} = [10(M) + 6.25(H) - 5(A) + S] \times L$$
>
> M = WEIGHT (KG)
> # LBS ÷ 2.2 = # KG
>
> H = HEIGHT (CM)
> # INCHES × 2.54 = # CM
>
> A = AGE
>
> S = SEX
> MALES ADD 5
> FEMALES SUBTRACT 161
>
> L = ACTIVITY LEVEL
>
> ___
>
> **ACTIVITY LEVEL (L)**
> SEDENTARY = BMR × 1.2
> LIGHTLY ACTIVE = BMR × 1.375
> MODERATELY ACTIVE = BMR × 1.55
> VERY ACTIVE = BMR × 1.725
> EXTRA ACTIVE = BMR × 1.9

Instead of digesting three large meals several hours apart, allow your body to burn food throughout the day by eating five or six small meals. Eat foods from a variety of groups. Take at least half of your calories from whole grains, fruits and vegetables. Try to eat some lean protein at each meal.

Be sure to get a little physical activity each day, even if it is just a half-hour walk after dinner. Add in some meditation and deep, mindful breathing to alleviate stress. Now you have the basics covered: food, energy, and oxygen. All three are vital for maintaining a healthy metabolism.

It might take longer than you like to see a weight loss with this method, but the loss you do attain will be a healthy and permanent one. Some

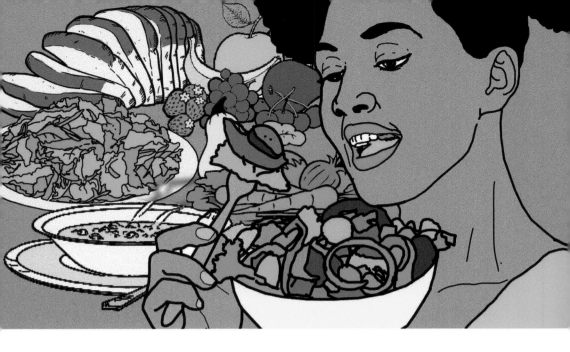

habitual dieters are able to speed up their metabolisms in weeks. Others take months. Your individual success will depend on age, genetics, and adherence to the plan.

> ### Remember
>
> **Diets slow down metabolism, but it can be repaired! Give your body small doses of fuel throughout the day, plus the movement and oxygen it needs. This is a simple, proven trick for getting your metabolism back on track.**

To better understand the reasoning behind this "eat more" trick, let us take a crash course in dieting and metabolism.

Everyone has a certain amount of calories that they must consume in order for their bodies to function properly. This is called the Basal Metabolic Rate (BMR). You can find BMR calculators online, or you can quickly estimate your BMR by using this simple system:

- 12 to 13 calories per pound of body weight will result in weight loss
- 15 to 16 calories per pound of body weight will result in weight maintenance
- 17 to 18 calories per pound of body weight will result in weight gain

NOTE: These estimates assume that you get a regular amount of physical activity each day. If you are completely sedentary or very active, your calorie requirements will vary. Use a BMR calculator that takes various activity levels into consideration.

Dieting can lower your BMR by 20 – 30%. Very low-calorie diets, also known as starvation diets, result in the most damage. A healthy, active 150-pound person needs approximately 2,200 calories per day to maintain their body weight. If that same person goes on a low-calorie diet, they will maintain their body weight on a mere 1,870 calories. Now, let us say that person decides to lose a few pounds. If the dieter has a healthy metabolism, they can lose weight by consuming 1,800 calories a day. But with a diet-damaged metabolism, that dieter will need to drop their daily calorie consumption to 1,260. That is bordering on dangerously low. Our 12-week weight loss plan on the LifestyleChangeWithApril will help you lose weight the healthy way by tracking your calories.

Chapter 7

A Practical Approach to Healthy Eating

> April, I've cut carbs from my diet and still no progress! I have 55kg to lose. Help!

I f you are overweight, you are not a bad person; you are simply overweight. But it is important to lose the extra pounds so you will look good, feel healthier and develop a sense of pride and self-esteem. Once you have lost the fat, you will need to maintain your weight. Most people pack on those extra pounds by eating the wrong things. Some others are just confused; they do not know what to eat. Changing these poor eating habits is the key to long-term success. Knowledge—along with the right food—is the key. Each one of us is born with a certain number of fat cells. The number of fat cells you possess depends on genetics.

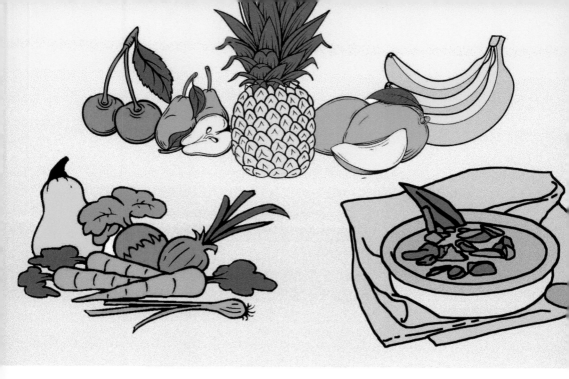

To guarantee a lifetime of weight-control success, you have to change the type of foods you eat, so that you ingest less fat and still get the vitamins, minerals, trace elements, protein, fat and carbohydrates your body needs to thrive. Extremely low-calorie diets may help you shed pounds quickly, but they will lead to failure in the long run. That is because humans are genetically protected against starvation. Have you ever heard the saying you are what you eat? This is somewhat true, because if you eat unhealthy foods you are prone to be an unhealthy person. The foods we ingest are extremely important to our ability to grow, function, and prevent illnesses. Therefore, if you value your health, you should learn as much about healthy eating as possible. My food nutritionist mother gave me a first hand experience of healthy eating with her freshly made soups, vegetables and fruits as snacks in my lunch boxes.

Asides weight loss, as a human being, you need food to survive and healthy eating is important throughout life. Children grow quite rapidly and this is due in part to the foods they eat. Foods contain nutrients that provide us not only with fuel to live our daily lives, but also with the very substances that build our bones, muscles, and organ tissues. Not getting enough of one nutrient or another can cause a variety of problems, including kwashiorkor. For pregnant and nursing moms, nutrition is important for many reasons. Your child depends on you for nutrients when they are developing as foetus. Once born, breast milk contains the nutrients a child needs to grow and develop properly. As we grow, so does our need for more substantial solid foods, however our bodies' need for proper nutrition never changes.

I have been running daily for over 4 years and my legs are pretty toned but this did not happen overnight. I also did not start running ten kilometres in a day. I started with brisk walking, to jogging, to running my first five-kilometre race and now looking forward to a marathon in a few months. I had to make running a habit with the intention to complete a marathon.

This drives home the truth of healthy eating. You will never be healthy, eating a salad once a week or drinking a smoothie once in a month. You have

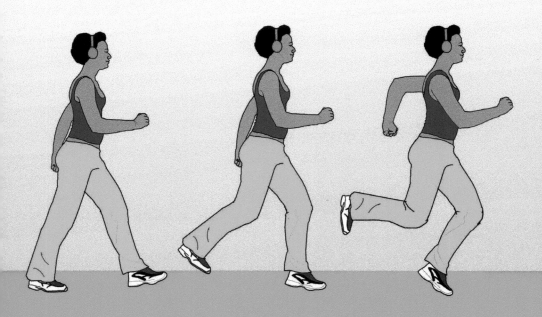

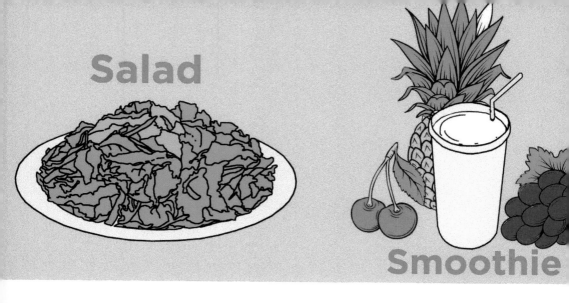

to make healthy eating a lifestyle if you want to obtain nutritional health or lose weight. A lot of people are on the 'fitfam' wagon because they feel it is trendy without necessarily making healthy eating a habit. Thus in a short period of time when temptations come, people fall right back into their old unhealthy eating habits.

What is a habit? According to Webster's dictionary a "habit" is "a behaviour pattern acquired by frequent repetition or physiologic exposure that shows itself in regularity or increased facility of performance." Can you see that if we simply apply this principle to healthy eating, we will be living our best lives? Bad eating habits are not developed overnight and would take

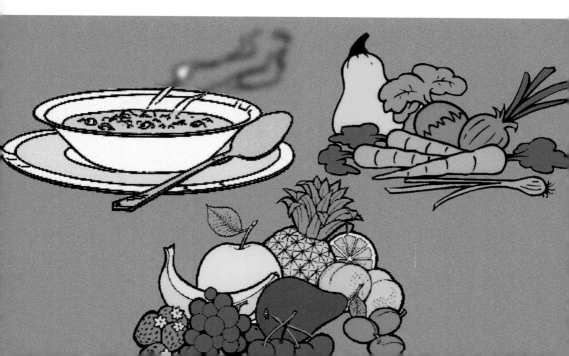

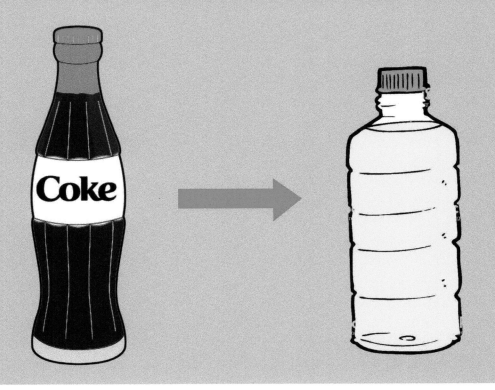

some time to change. For most people, these habits began forming when they were teens. How do you tell an adult who is used to drinking a bottle of coke with every meal to replace that with a bottle of water? This is one of the reasons many adults have a hard time breaking bad eating habits; because these habits have been a part of their lifestyle for many years.

So many people think that healthy eating is boring. Far from it, eating healthy is not boring or tasteless. I think that one reason people feel this way is because most of the commercial ads we see promote junk foods while only a small percentage of food advertising is done for fruits, vegetables, grains and beans. Thus if there was more nutritional education, more and more people would find eating healthy to be pleasurable and tasty. I will be sharing my healthy recipes in my next book. You can pre-order here.

So, how can one eat healthy and clean, without starving? When we drastically cut back our food intake, the brain thinks the body is starving, and in an effort to preserve life, it slows the metabolism. Soon the pounds stop coming off. Consequently, we grow hungry and uncomfortable and then eat more. And then the diet fails.

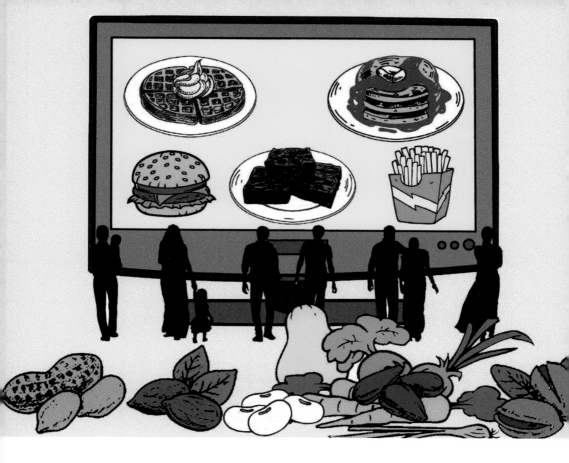

How can you compensate for this metabolic slow-down? The answer is that you have to change the nutritional composition of the foods you eat. You will have to cut down on total calories—that is absolutely basic to weight loss. More important, however, is reducing the percentage of total calories you are getting from fat. That is how you will avoid starvation panic in your system. At the same time, you reduce the amount of fat in your food, replacing it with safe, low calorie, nutrient-rich plant foods. This will convince your brain that your body is getting all the nutrition it needs.

In fact, you will be able to eat more food and feel more satisfied while consuming fewer calories and fats. Vegetable foods break down slowly in your stomach, making you feel full longer, and they are rich in vitamins, minerals, trace elements, carbohydrates and protein for energy and muscle-building. This allows your body to burn off its excess stored fat. Let me introduce you to a healthy shopping basket.

A healthy shopping basket should have the following items:

Grains:	
Vegetables:	Asparagus, Avocado, Beets, Bell peppers (green, red, orange, yellow) Broccoli, Brussels sprouts, Cabbage (green, red) Carrots, Corn, sweet yellow, Green beans, Kale, Lettuce/greens, Mushrooms, Onions (green, red, white, yellow) Peas, Radishes, Squash (summer, winter) Spinach, Sweet potatoes, Swiss chard, Tomatoes
Fruits:	Apples, Apricots, Bananas, Blueberries, Cantaloupe, Cherries, Cranberries, Figs, Grapes, Grapefruit, Kiwifruit, Mangoes, Oranges, Peaches, Pineapples, Plums, Prunes (dried plums), Raisins, Raspberries, Strawberries, Watermelon
Dairy / Dairy Alternatives:	Cheese (Low fat), Eggs, Milk (Low Fat), Almond Milk, Soymilk, Yogurt
Fish:	Cod, Tuna, Sardines, Salmon, Shrimps, Mackerel, Scallops
Poultry:	Chicken and Turkey
Nuts/Seeds and Legumes:	Almonds, Black Eyed Beans, Chickpeas, Kidney Beans, Lentils, Peanut Butter, Peanuts, Pine Nuts, Pinto Beans, Pistachios, Pumpkn Seeds, Sunflower Seeds, Sesame Seeds, Soybeans, Tofu, Walnuts
Oils:	Canola Oil, Coconut Oil, Sunflower Oil

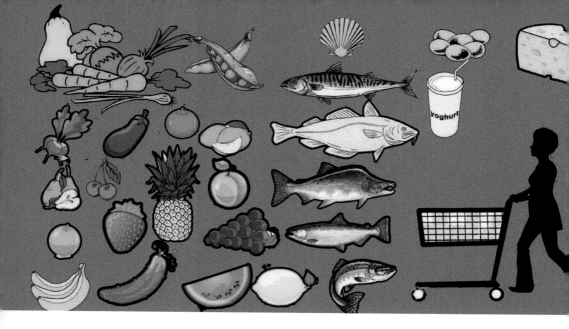

So what are fat burning foods?

Each one of the following foods is clinically proven to promote weight loss and they are my absolutely favourites. These foods go a step beyond simply adding no fat to your system, they possess special properties that add zip to your system and help your body melt away unhealthy pounds. These incredible foods can suppress your appetite for junk food and keep your body running smoothly with clean fuel and efficient energy. You can include these foods in any sensible weight-loss plan. They give your body the extra metabolic kick that it needs to shave off weight quickly.

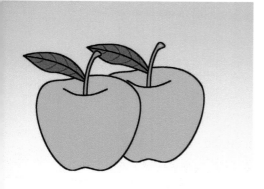

Apples

Who does not like or eat apples? These marvels of nature deserve their reputation for keeping the doctor away when you eat one a day. And now, it seems, they can help you melt the fat away, too. First of all, they elevate your blood glucose levels in a safe, gentle manner and keep them up

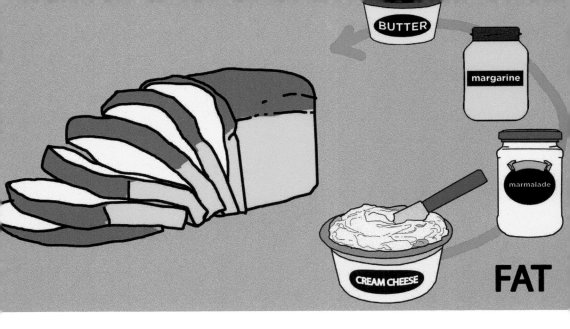

longer than most foods. The practical effect of this is to leave you feeling satisfied longer, researchers say. An average size apple provides only 81 calories and has no sodium, saturated fat or cholesterol. You will also get the added health benefits of lowering the level of cholesterol already in your blood as well as lowering your blood pressure.

Whole grain bread

Bread is not the problem. It is the other things that escort it on its journey to the stomach—the butter, margarine, marmalade or cream cheese—that are fattening, not the bread itself. I will say this as often as needed—fat is fattening. It is even the base word of "fattening". If you do not believe that, ponder this—a gram of carbohydrate has four calories; a gram of protein, four, and a gram of fat, nine. So which of these is really fattening? Bread, a natural source of fibre and complex carbohydrates, is okay for weight loss. Studies with my husband show some kinds

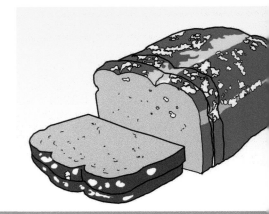

of bread actually reduce the appetite. So the key is eating dark, rich, high-fibre breads such as, whole wheat, mixed grain, oatmeal and others. The average slice of whole grain bread contains only 60 to 70 calories, is rich in complex carbohydrates—the best, steadiest fuel you can give your body—and delivers surprising amount of protein.

Coffee

Please go easy on this one. We have all heard about potential dangers of caffeine, including anxiety and insomnia, so moderation is the key. The caffeine in coffee can speed up your metabolism. This makes sense, since caffeine is a stimulant. Studies show it can help you burn more calories than normal, perhaps up to 10 per cent more. For safety sake, it is best to limit your intake to a single cup in the morning and one in the afternoon. Add only skimmed milk to it and try doing without sugar—many people learn to love it that way.

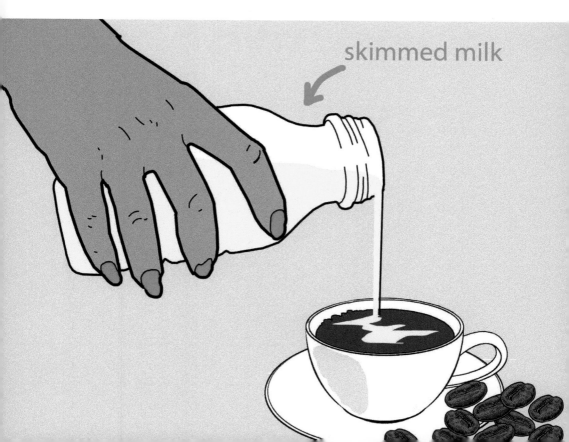

Grapefruit

An average sized grapefruit has 74 calories; delivers a whopping 15 grams of pectin (the special fibre linked to lowering cholesterol and fat); is high in vitamin C and potassium and is free of fat and sodium. It is rich in natural galacturonic acid, which adds to its potency as a fat and cholesterol fighter. The additional benefit here is assistance in the battle against atherosclerosis—hardening of the arteries—and reduces your chances of developing heart disease. Try sprinkling it with cinnamon rather than sugar to take away some of the tart taste.

Peppers

Hot, spicy chilli peppers also known as scotch bonnet are fantastic for weight loss. A mere three grams of chilli peppers were added to a meal consisting of 766 total calories. Peppers are astonishingly rich in vitamins A and C, abundant in calcium, phosphorus, iron and magnesium, high in fibre, free of fat, low in sodium and have just 24 calories per cup.

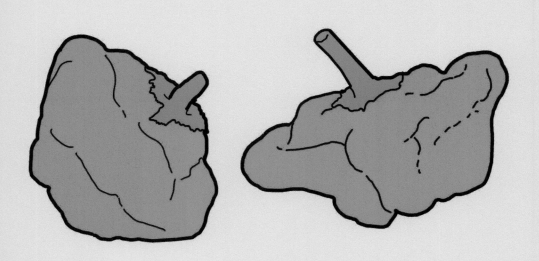

Potatoes

We've got to be kidding, right? Wrong. Potatoes have developed the same "fattening" rap as bread, and it is unfair on the poor little yummy roots. A great source of fibre and potassium, they lower cholesterol and protect against strokes and heart disease.

Rice

A cup of cooked rice (150 grams) contains about 178 calories – approximately one-third the number of calories found in an equivalent amount of beef or cheese. And remember, whole grain rice is much better for you than white rice.

Soups

Soup is good for you! Maybe not the canned varieties from the store – but old-fashioned, homemade soup promotes weight loss. Naturally, the type of soup you eat makes a difference. Cream soups or those made of beef or pork are not your best bets. You will find a great recipe on Detox with April Guide.

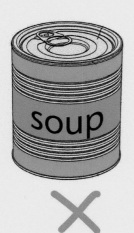

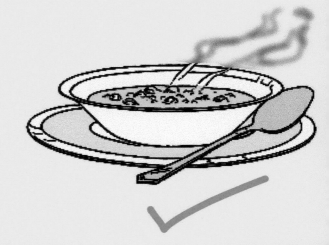

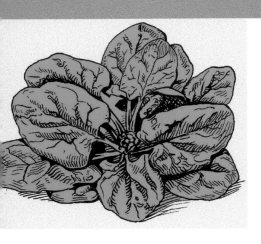

Snacking Strategies

Intermittent snacking can lead to grams of calories that are difficult to shed. Most snacks pack on unhealthy carbs that are difficult to lose. Look around you; how many snacks are healthy? Ask yourself, when last did you snack on anything with healthy vitamins? Wait, it is not an outright cancellation. You can work with snacks on this journey; just in the right portion and at the right time. You can still snack and remain healthy! Yes! Here are some strategies to snacking the healthy way.

Don't need it, don't buy it!

There's no visitor that is coming to greet you in a few weeks that would need that bucket of ice cream in your fridge. If you do not have junk food lying

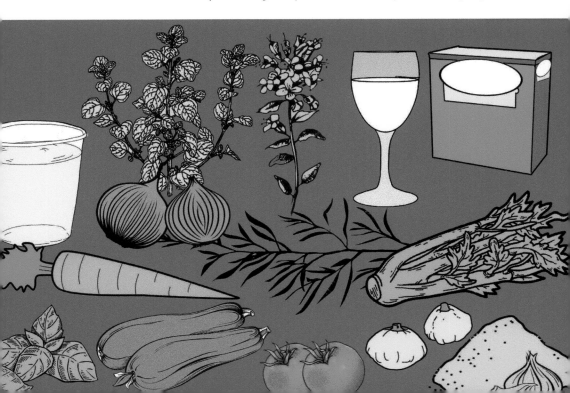

around, the sight of it will not tempt you, so do not even bring it home. After all, you cannot eat what is not there. We are all humans and the more temptations we have around, the farther we are from reaching our goals.

Don't skip meals!

You are only going on a journey of self-deprivation not weight loss if you skip your meals. Skipping meals may seem like a good way to cut calories, but in fact this just makes you so hungry later in the day and you go out of proportions with your servings or succumb to a junk meal.

Snack mindfully not mindlessly!

If you cannot watch your favourite TV show without a bowl of popcorn in sight or browse the internet without chewing on something, this is mindless eating and it can sabotage your progress. Get a substitute to these snacks, a cup of tea would do no harm and if you must snack, watch the portions.

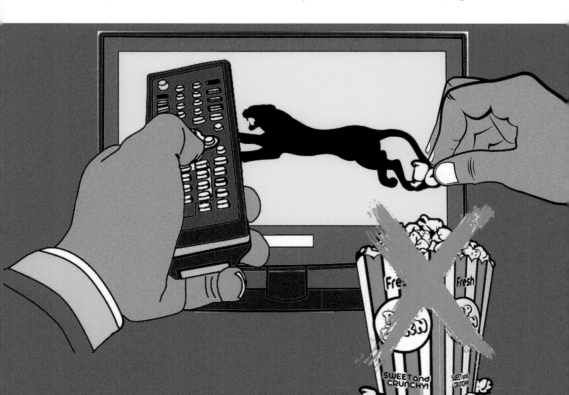

Zero in on hunger.

Before you snack, ask yourself, "Am I truly hungry?" Many of us mistake emotions, such as stress and fatigue, for hunger. Sometimes, all you need is a glass of water, make sure you are not confusing hunger with thirst. Drink a glass of water; then wait 10 to 15 minutes. If you are still hungry, have a healthful snack; like a handful of nuts, apple and peanut butter, GuiltFreeKitchen muffins or a bowl of sugar-free popcorn.

Identify your cravings.

If you want a snack but you are not hungry, then why are you eating it? Ask yourself how you are feeling at that particular time. Lonely? Bored? Stressed at work? Stuck in traffic? Will food solve this problem? Trust me; eating a burger would not solve the problem of a petty boss. Why not call your best friend or take a long walk away from the stressor than resorting to food? You can also listen to some music, or choose another simple activity that might distract you or boost your mood. And if the craving persists, have a bite and give the rest to the poor! If you are craving chocolate, for example, eat one small square and savour it for hours! LOL! I'm just saying, it is important that you snack on what you are craving rather than deny the craving and then end up eating a double portion of it.

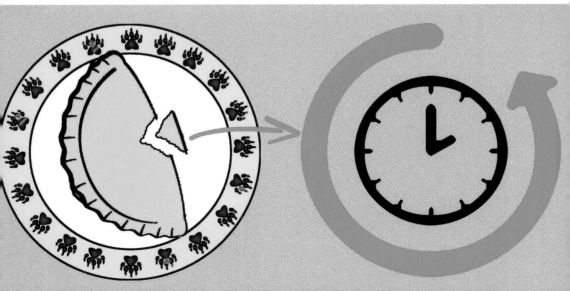

Chapter 8

Eating for a Sustained Weight Loss

You have probably heard this a lot of time 'eat clean, to lose weight!' You have probably wondered what the magic behind eating to lose weight is all about. Do you really eat to lose weight? Yes. However, to start losing weight the right away, you will need to know the scientific principles behind weight loss. Let's start by learning how many calories you actually need each day.

Your Basal Metabolic Rate, or BMR, dictates how many calories your body needs to perform its functions for the day. This number is the bare minimum; it tells you how many calories your body needs to simply survive and carry out natural processes. If you are an active person, you will require more calories than your BMR suggests. The sum of your BMR plus the calories you burn during daily activities is your Total Energy Expenditure, or TEE.

There are various formulas you can use to figure out an appropriate number of calories for weight loss. The most widely used is the Harris-Benedict formula, which considers your age, gender, height, and current weight to come up with a suitable number of calories. Here is an example of this formula in action:

Men: BMR = 66 + (13.7 X wt in kg) + (5 X ht in cm) – (6.8 X age in years)

Women: BMR = 655 + (9.6 X wt in kg) + (1.8 X ht in cm) – (4.7 X age in years)

(For calculation purposes, 1 inch = 2.54 cm and 1 kilogram = 2.2 lbs.)

Example:

A 35 year old female who stands 5'4" (163 cm) tall and weighs 130 pounds (59 kilos) would use the following equation:

655 + 566 + 293 – 165 = 1,349.

The woman in the example would need 1,349 calories a day just to lie around in bed and keep her organs functioning. If that number seems small, it is because we have not taken this woman's activity level into consideration.

Activity multipliers work as such:

Sedentary people (office jobs, no real exercise) multiply their BMR by 1.2.

Lightly active people (exercise 1-3 times per week) multiply their BMR by 1.35.

Moderately active people (exercise 4-5 times per week) multiply their BMR by 1.55.

Highly active people (sports or hard exercise most days) multiply their BMR by 1.725.

Extremely active people (hard exercise every day) multiply their BMR by 1.9.

Let us revisit the woman in our example. We will assume she works a desk job and is sedentary most days of the week. Even at such a low activity level, she would expend extra calories walking around, driving to and from work, typing, and fidgeting at her desk.

Her BMR (1,349) multiplied by her sedentary activity level (1.2) reveals that she needs about 1,619 calories each day to maintain her current weight. If she started exercising just 2 or 3 days each week, her daily calorie requirement would increase to 1,821.

So how do these numbers help you lose weight? Easy: To lose a pound of fat each week, you must burn 3,500 more calories than you consume. In order to lose a pound of fat, the woman in our example would need to eat 1,119 calories a day if sedentary, or 1,321 a day if lightly active.

Too much Mathematics? Let's break it down. Once you calculate your BMR and you know what you need to eat in terms of the calories, then you can easily know how much you need to burn daily to lose weight. If April burns 3,500 calories weekly and she eats 1,300 calories daily, she's already

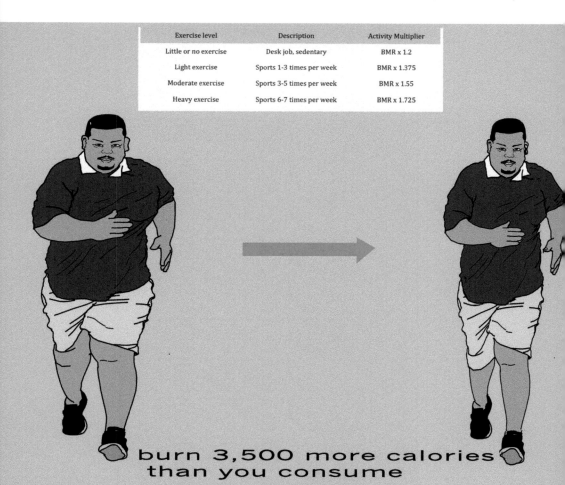

Exercise level	Description	Activity Multiplier
Little or no exercise	Desk job, sedentary	BMR x 1.2
Light exercise	Sports 1-3 times per week	BMR x 1.375
Moderate exercise	Sports 3-5 times per week	BMR x 1.55
Heavy exercise	Sports 6-7 times per week	BMR x 1.725

burn 3,500 more calories than you consume

in a deficit of what she is burning versus eating. With this, she will lose 1 pound a week. It is very much easier to lose weight through diet and physical activity than through diet alone. They go hand in hand like bread and butter haha! And you see results faster, with the amount of energy you put in daily.

Many of us have many excuses for our sedentary lifestyles. We work too hard, cannot afford gym memberships, have too many demands on our time, or just plain don't like to exercise. If you hate exercising, it is probably because you are not getting the right kind of exercise. You really have to find an activity that you enjoy and stick to it as a routine. Some people are perfectly happy running on a treadmill day in and day out, but there are many more who dread the monotony. For me, I love to jump ropes and running outdoors. For days I cannot make it to the gym, I get my workouts done at home in my garden with my son, Bryan watching.

If boredom is keeping you from getting a healthy amount of cardio, mix up your routine with some fun activities. Group sports like basketball and flag softball burn far more calories per hour than a treadmill, and they

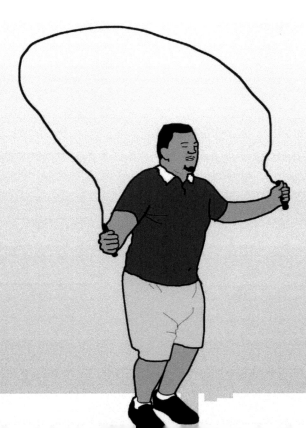

are fun and social to boot. Call up some friends, or visit your local activity centre to sign up for an amateur sports league.

Swimming is another great way to burn calories. Jump in the pool and paddle around, then jog as fast as you can in the shallow end. The water provides enough resistance to kick your metabolism into high gear. If you have a local beach, brisk walking on the sand will burn more calories than walking on pavement.

As a mom, you have to learn to balance your daily life to fit in some workouts. Kids also provide opportunities for calorie burning. If you have a baby, contact your local stroller club to go on walks with other new parents or take the stroll on your own. You can keep an eye on your little one while you get in shape. If your child is older, they will appreciate some one-on-one time spent tossing a football, shooting hoops, or just swinging and sliding on the playground. These activities help you burn calories while you bond with your child.

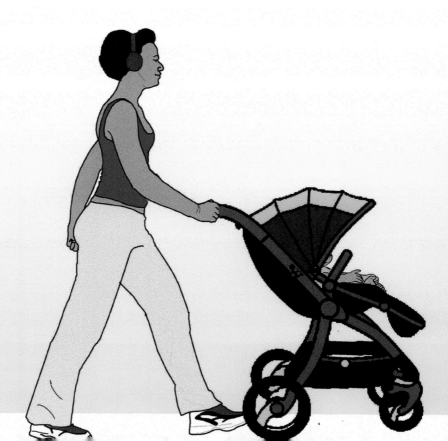

If you have a garden, you have got a calorie-burning goldmine. Lawn work, including mowing the grass and planting shrubs and saplings, is a great way to firm up and lose pounds. Weeding, pruning, picking flowers and vegetables, and laying sod are all calorie-burning activities. Spend an hour a day working on your landscaping, and you will soon see the results in your yard— and on the scale.

Maybe you are an animal lover. Try walking your dog in the evening, or taking the neighbours' dogs for a walk. Take your pet to the park for some Frisbee action. Saddle up a horse and go for a relaxing trail ride. Don't have a pet of your own? Try volunteering at a ranch or animal shelter. Caring for and cleaning up after the animals is a rewarding act that enriches their lives and helps you stay in shape.

You are on your way home and there is this long traffic? Get out of the car and start walking. If the traffic moves, you may join your car—or bus— again. If not, you may just turn the ride into a long walk home. You could walk, as though you are strolling, you could jog a little or run-walk. If it is a short trip, you may still get home in time and you would have burnt some calories along the way. You can also dance to your favourite Naija music, anything to keep you moving.

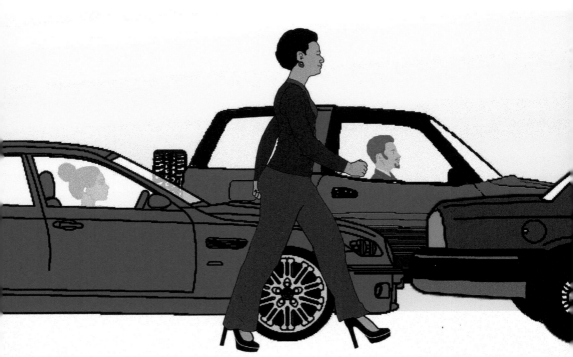

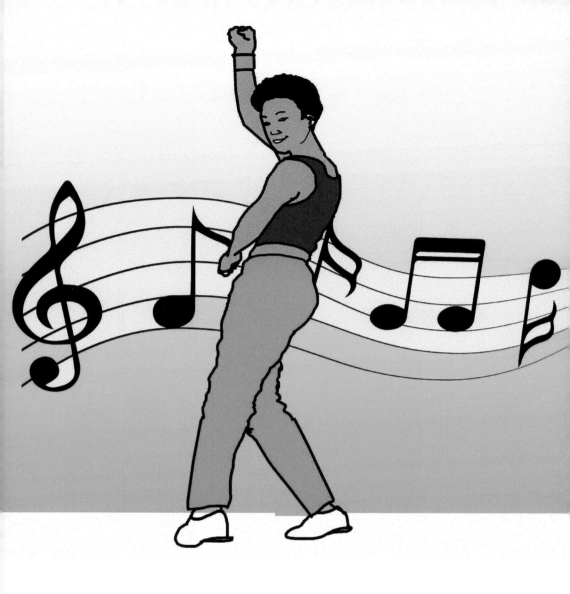

Chapter 9

Tips to Burn Calories and Stay Motivated

Good morning fithive! It's a brand new week!! Rise and Shine!!! I hope you're all ready to hit your goals this week? I am o! The run challenge is still ON and my goal this week is to complete my race! The abs challenge is still on and my goal this week is to double my reps. Where it says 10 push-ups, I'm pushing to do 20. If you haven't completed or started the RunWithApril challenge, get to it! We have 7 weeks left! If you're still struggling with your meals, continue to submit your meals as a collage at the end of the day and I'll review for you. Please be honest with this task so I can correct the little things that can be detrimental to your weight loss progress...if you're not losing weight and burning loads of calories — it's the food and you need to make a conscious effort to eat clean daily to see any progress. I pray that the Lord will guide our steps this week and make ways for us in all we do. Have a good day and week guys! Love you

April, please excuse me this week. I have a lot going on and I don't see exercise showing up.

Really, Tomi? What's taking all your time?

It's summer break. My toddlers are home plus this baby isn't sleeping all night yet. She wakes up for at least 4 times before the day breaks and I'm not even exaggerating! I also have a final thesis to submit by the weekend. Hubby is away tomorrow, no one to assist. I'm just tired, maybe I should take a break from this fit life. It's not for me at the moment. Please don't quote Philippians 4:13 today April.

But you have 20kg left to hit your goal? Don't you think…

April…

Okay, call me. Let's talk this out. You will be fine; you're on the right path.

Weight loss is not a walk in the park. Though it may involve some running, it is not a 100-metre dash. It takes patience. It takes commitment. For some, it is a lesson in persistence. For many, it is not the destination; it is about the journey, the process. A lifestyle does not change immediately. It took some decades to become who you are today; how does one change that in weeks? So, this journey needs a healthy dose of motivation. You get to some bus-stops and you just want to sit down there and wait but the goal is ahead.

It is pretty easy to feel gung-ho about your diet when you start out. It is something new, you are hopeful and enthusiastic, and you might even be looking forward to your new way of eating and exercising. Fast-forward two weeks, and you might find a different story entirely. You have gotten bored with your daily menu, the exercises seem like a chore, and perhaps you have even fallen off the wagon completely. Finding the initial motivation can be a challenge, but staying motivated may even be more difficult. Here are some ways you can sustain your enthusiasm until you reach the finish line.

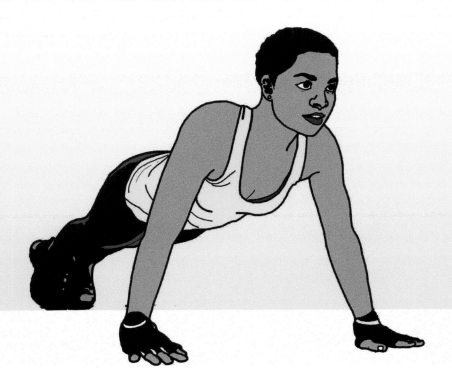

Set Small Milestones

For the sake of this example, let us say you need to lose 30 pounds. That sounds daunting! The goal might seem more manageable if you break it down into smaller milestones. For example, you could set yourself the goal of losing one pound in a week. If you stick to the plan, you can almost certainly reach that goal. Then you will only have 29 more milestones to go, and a sense of accomplishment to help you pass those milestones.

Treat Yourself Often

Humans are wired to love rewards. Personal achievement might be enough to keep some people going, but the rest of us need tangible rewards to keep moving forward. These rewards do not need to be expensive, but they do need to be motivational. For example, let us imagine you have reached your first milestone—one pound gone in one week. You could reward yourself with a guilt-free evening to goof off and play video

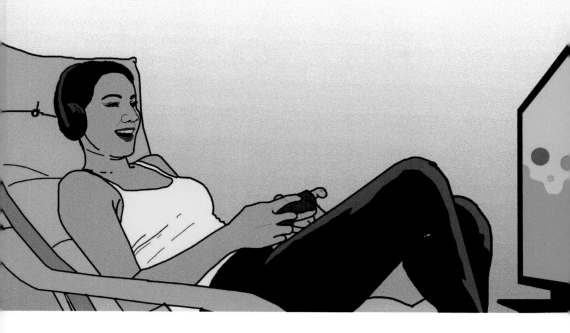

games, rent a movie you have wanted to see, or have an at-home spa session complete with a homemade facial and a do-it-yourself pedicure. Special milestones, such as the loss of 10 pounds, deserve larger treats! Get creative, and come up with several ideas. To make it fun. Little things can make it exciting and fun… I like buying a new pair of sneakers, or a new pair of leggings, changing my playlist, finding a good show to reward myself.

Should you use food as a weight loss reward? The concept is pretty controversial. Experts warn against it, but some dieters say it works for them. The bottom line is that you have to set up a reward system that will motivate you to keep going. If that means indulging in a hot fudge sundae, then eat the sundae. It is far better to have those extra calories than to give up on your diet because you feel deprived. Just be careful. If you tend to eat for comfort, the taste of a sundae could send you into a binge. Some dieters find it easier to stay on track by rewarding themselves with non-edible treats.

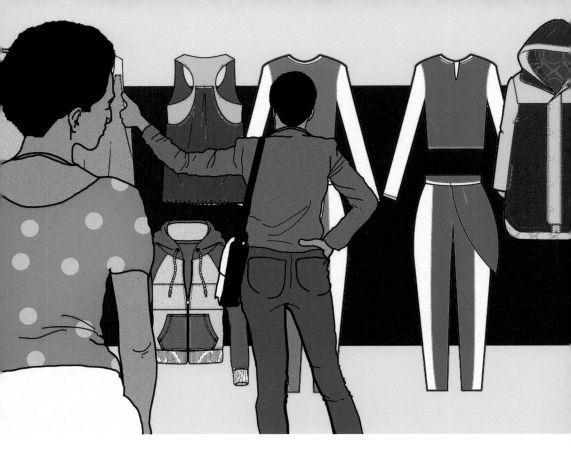

Find What Motivates You

Why do you want to lose weight? Many of us would answer with safe responses, like "I want to do it for my health", or "I want to fit into my old clothes again." These might be 100 per cent true, but for many dieters, that is not the whole story. Be brutally honest with yourself. Even if you think the truth is ugly, go ahead and take a personal inventory of all the reasons why you want to lose weight. Do you want to be considered a hottie? Do you want your exes to kick themselves for letting you go? Do you want to be able to wear more risqué clothing styles? Do you want to avoid getting jowly as you age? Some of those reasons might sound vain and selfish, but many dieters use them as personal motivators. If they help you stick to your diet and fitness plan, use them.

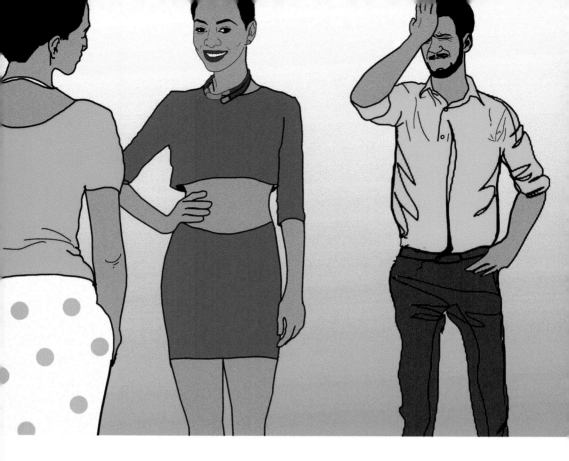

Keep a Journal

Studies have shown that dieters who keep food journals are more likely to lose weight and keep it off. It is good to track the calories in the journal but you can keep a journal to track more than just your calories. Start writing down your moods, level of hunger, and thoughts about your weight loss journey. Seeing everything in print can help you identify situations that make you want to eat. A journal can also help you discover patterns in your eating, like skimping on breakfast and subsequently overeating at lunchtime. You can also use a journal to plan your milestones and rewards. Seeing your next reward spelled out in ink can keep you from giving in to a temporary urge to binge.

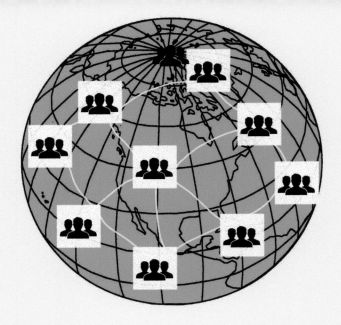

Share with Others

There is no need to go through your weight loss alone. The internet has brought together millions of people who want to lose weight. They have formed communities, meet-up groups, and social networking sites. Don't be shy; many of these people face the same hardships and struggles as you do. Jump right in and introduce yourself. Ask questions from long-time members. Share every little victory and setback, and congratulate and comfort others when they do the same. You might find that joining a community keeps you accountable not only to yourself, but to your new friends as well. You can also share your experiences with April Laugh.

Chapter 10

Weight Loss on Holiday

That sentence seems confusing: is my weight loss on a holiday or am I attempting to lose weight while on holiday? Either way, both ideas sound "somehow" or "one kain" as we say in Nigeria. They are ironic. How can your weight loss be on holiday? How can you be attempting to lose weight when you are supposed to be holidaying? It is not as complicated. In this chapter, we will learn how to go on a holiday, get all the fun, all the rest, the great food—and every other thing that comes with a holiday—and not gain weight. Yes!

Few months ago, my family and I were in Prague for the summer holiday and it was so much fun! We travel all the time and like you, I want to go on holiday without thinking about counting calories or my meal plan. When we go on vacation, we do not waste our time or energy worrying about calories. We eat what we want and we drink what we want, relaxing and enjoying ourselves to the fullest extent possible. That does not mean that all of the food that we eat is unhealthy, it just means that we do not allow ourselves to overthink it

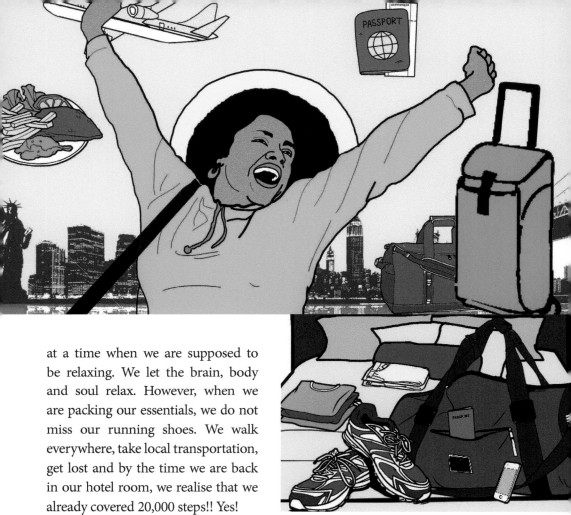

at a time when we are supposed to be relaxing. We let the brain, body and soul relax. However, when we are packing our essentials, we do not miss our running shoes. We walk everywhere, take local transportation, get lost and by the time we are back in our hotel room, we realise that we already covered 20,000 steps!! Yes!

With food, we try new dishes. However, we ensure that we eat loads of protein and vegetables with minimal carbs as we would if we were home. You should have an idea of what your portions should look like by now. We do not eat a lot of bread or burgers or those high and mighty meals. *Laughing out loud!* So by the time we are home, after getting our taste buds familiarised with food from different parts of the world, it is easy to jump right back into meal prepping and working out without adding any weight. And if we did add weight, trust me, it is so inconsequential and really not worth stressing over. As long as you are able to get home and snap right back into your normal habits of eating clean and working out on a regular basis, there is no reason to spoil your vacation obsessing over what might be happening with your weight scale.

Do not forget to stay hydrated when you are away. I have noticed water is usually more expensive in hotels. *Kiss my teeth.* So, we always try to buy from stores to last us all through the number of days we would be vacationing for. And yes, we grab a bottle anytime we are stepping out. Water should not be something anyone would think about before drinking!

Weight loss might be your number one goal, but eating healthy and working out makes you feel good, and you want to feel good on vacation. So allowing yourself cheat meals and cheat days while away is fine, but you also want to fuel your body in a way that makes you feel your best. Finding a combination of taking care of yourself on vacation without obsessing about calories and weight loss or gain is most ideal.

Follow these simple rules and you will be able to relax and truly enjoy yourself while away.

1.) Earn Your Feast

So few weeks before travelling, I always make sure that I burn excess calories. You will think I am going for a marathon! So for instance, if on a regular day, I burn 500 calories, increase that to 1,000, two weeks before I pack my bag. This will give me a calorie deficit in advance, before the trip.

2.) Chew While You Chop

If you rented an apartment instead of the regular hotel booking, you'll need to shop for plenty of snacks. To avoid nibbling, pop a piece of gum to occupy your mouth when you are in the kitchen so you can save those calories for the treats you will really enjoy. When grabbing a pack, reach for spearmint or peppermint rather than a sweet or fruity flavour.

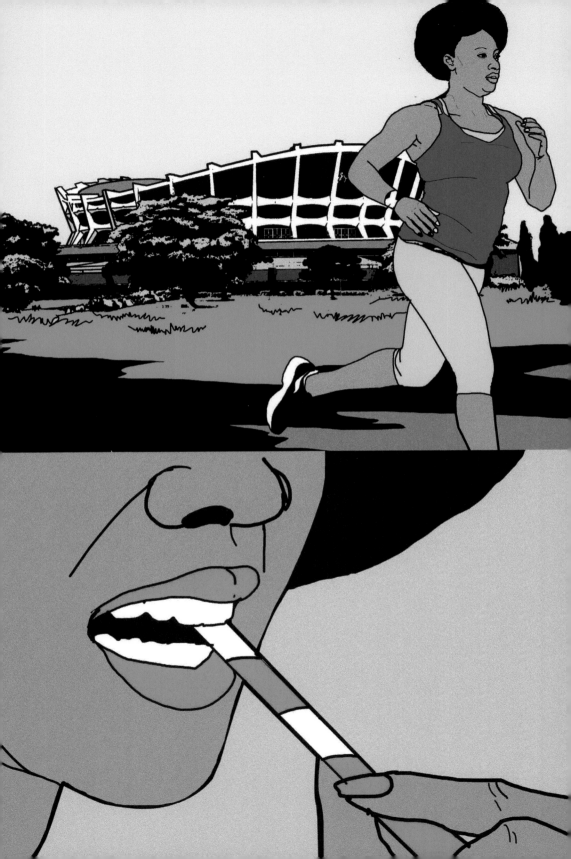

3.) Be a Picky Eater

With some advance planning, even the most decadent buffet can become a diet too. The first step: survey your options. Before you belly up to the table, peruse the entire spread so you know exactly what you have to choose from. Then go back and, instead of tasting everything, help yourself to just the three or four things that catch your eye. And because it takes at least 20 minutes for a feeling of fullness to set in, swap memories with your sister or slowly sip a glass of water before going back to the table for a second helping or dessert.

4.) Seize Some ZZZ's

The last time I was away in Barcelona, one of the unforgettable experiences I took from there was the ability to sleep for hours! My gosh! My husband and I made it compulsory not to step out of our hotel, just to actually REST. Between sight seeing, holiday shopping, and eating out, sleep may be the first thing that gets cut from your endless to-do list. But skimping on shut-eye can do more than create under-eye circles. The more exhausted you are, the hungrier you will likely feel; and the more you eat (mindlessly), the more the weight you may actually gain.

To make sure you get plenty of sleep, set an alarm for an hour before your usual bedtime as a reminder to start winding down. If you cannot stop ruminating about the 1,001 things you still have to accomplish before you leave, make a list before turning in and keep it on your bedside table. Putting your worries and tasks on paper will help you clear your mind—so you can start dreaming about how you will look in that bodycon dress you bought from Zara! Haha!

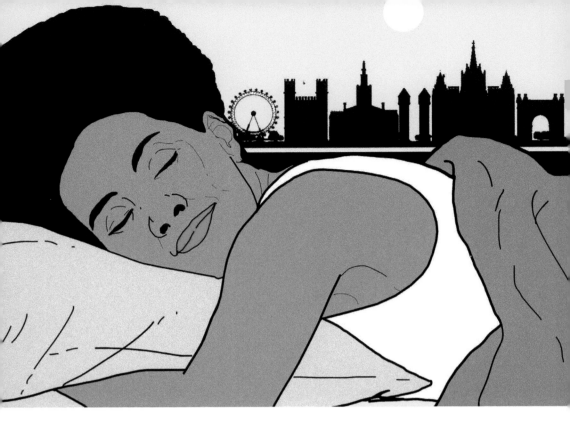

5.) Take Dainty Bites

You know better than to shovel in your food, but even the average mouthful may be your dietary downfall. According to a new study in the *American Journal of Clinical Nutrition*,[4] people who took bites about the size of a tablespoon ate 25 per cent more at a meal than those who took teaspoon-size ones. Avoid taking a full fork or spoonful; your food should cover less than half the utensil. Also, reach for the smallest plate you can find. Call it a game of tricks—your brain tricks your hand which now tricks your stomach. In the end, the tricks have their effects: number of calories ingested reduces and your body is glad!

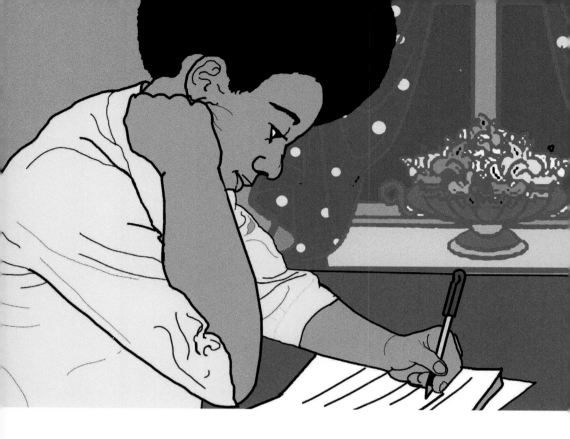

6.) Start Skinny Sipping

Whoa! Whoa! Whoa! What is that? With just 123 calories for a 5-ounce glass, wine is a calorie bargain compared to other alcoholic beverages, like gin and tonic (164 calories), buttered rum–spiced cider (275 calories), and eggnog (321 calories). It is not only your food that you check the amount of calories your body packs on when ingested, even drinks—well except water. If you're in the mood for a cocktail, feel free— but have only one alcoholic beverage before switching to a lower-calorie drink, like iced tea or sparkling water with a twist of lemon or lime. So yes, it is a holiday and you are having the time of your life, watch the alcohol, and the calories that come in the bottle.

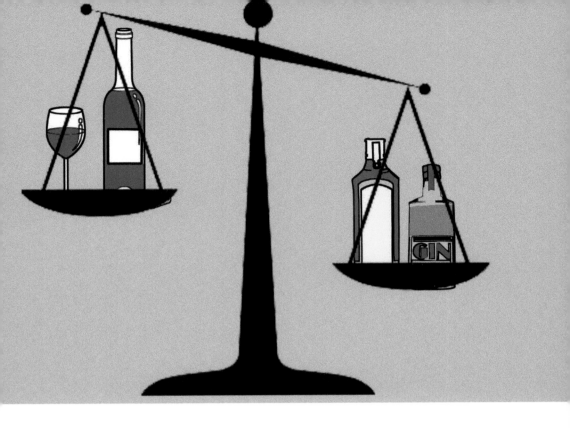

7.) Remain Active

It is supposed to be a holiday right? It is important to keep your body active even though all that you want to do is relax. And yes, not only the physical body should be active, get your mind engaged. So, find a mixture of activities. While shopping for activities to pack on your trip—it is not only clothes you shop for—consider things that are also intellectually stimulating. Find activities that teach you something new about the place, the people, and their history. And take things slowly. Pause. Think. Breathe. Ask questions. Find directions. Visit friends. Challenge yourself. Set a milestone. Break your rules. Make new ones. Learn a new word, slang, a new phrase. All these things make your holiday experience richer, fuller, leading to a better and different you. Though looking at it, these may not look like they add up to a great body but remember a great physical body is connected to a great mind. So, while you are nourishing the physical body while on holiday, find different ways to also allow your mind luxuriate in a new experience.

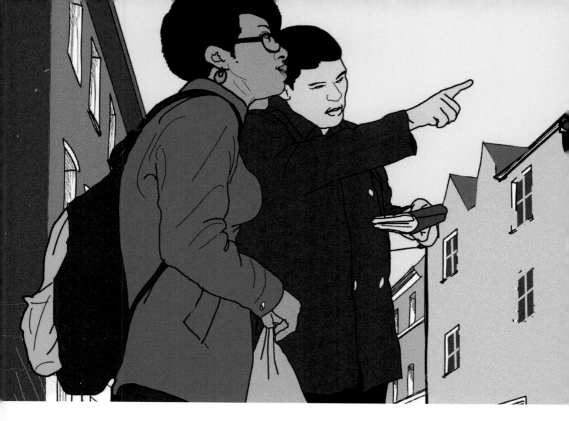

Your body will thank you for it. And after the holiday, the new glow may be unexplainable.

   If you still gain weight after your holiday, the best way to get out of the 'feeling full' rut is to have a detox. You will find our *Detox with April Guide* attached to this book helpful!

Chapter 11

Healthy Pregnancy

> *My mum and aunt discouraged me from exercising because I am TTC. I really need to lose between 10-15kg. I gained some weight when I got married this year but I keep hearing stuff like 'if you're exercising and you conceive, it won't stay. You're stressing yourself, and stress inhibits conception. Really how healthy is it? Can I resume exercises, because I've been TTC for 5 months? I honestly don't like the fact that some of my clothes don't fit anymore. Is it too late?*

No, it is not too late! There is no reason to give up exercise before pregnancy. This plays a huge role in your overall health and wellness and according to research, can help prepare your body for conception and pregnancy. The only exception is, as we all know too much of a good thing can be, well, too much for your body when you are trying to conceive. Super-intense exercise during pre-conception can alter your menstrual cycle and even halt ovulation.

I am a woman and a bit of a fitness freak who exercises a lot. Over the years, I fell in love with running and weight lifting. Running because it is good cardio and weights because I love my body toned to the gods! If you exercised regularly before pregnancy comes, continue your programme, with modifications as you need them.

Running is an excellent cardiovascular activity; and it is a guaranteed way to get your blood pumping. I ran 150km within the first six weeks of my first trimester and when I noticed that my runs were wearing me out, I toned down the frequency, pace, and duration. I didn't stop running.

Weight lifting is also a great form of exercise. It builds muscle tone and bone strength — both of which will keep you in top shape before and during pregnancy. Like I always say, no woman should lift anything lighter than her purse. You don't have to buff up like a Warrior Princess by lifting massive tons of heavy metal. Lift medium weights with more repetitions or focus on resistance exercises that use your own body weight (lunges, squats, crunches, and push-ups).

Adopting a habit of regular exercise before conceiving should not come from the woman alone. This should be a joint effort with your partner as it has proven benefits for increasing both fertility and ovulation, and strengthening the body for the normal pregnancy and delivery. Studies have shown that proper exercise can help increase sperm count, so ask your partner to work out with you which will also increase your time together. So what can you do while you are trying to conceive? Below are some fitness tips:

Start Early: It is more efficient if you stay fit before you get pregnant to keep your body healthy and ready for all changes you will experience. It is also advisable to be on a healthy weight so if you are overweight, you might consider losing the weight and staying on a healthy diet.

Do not Lose Track: There are days when we do not feel like exercising, it happens to the best of trainers. This might not just be you being lazy; a monotonous exercise routine can also cause this. To avoid this, switch things up and adopt different forms of exercises such as swimming, walking, aerobics and dance classes. Have fun while at it.

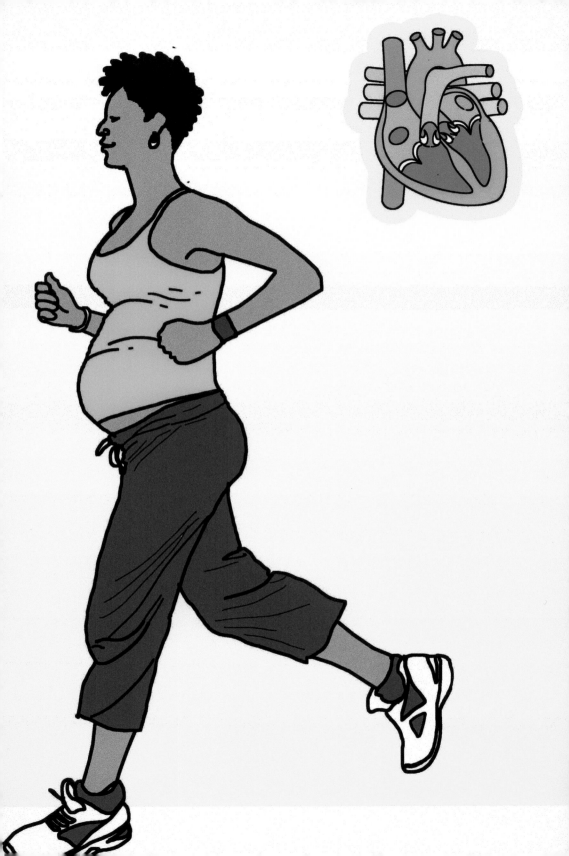

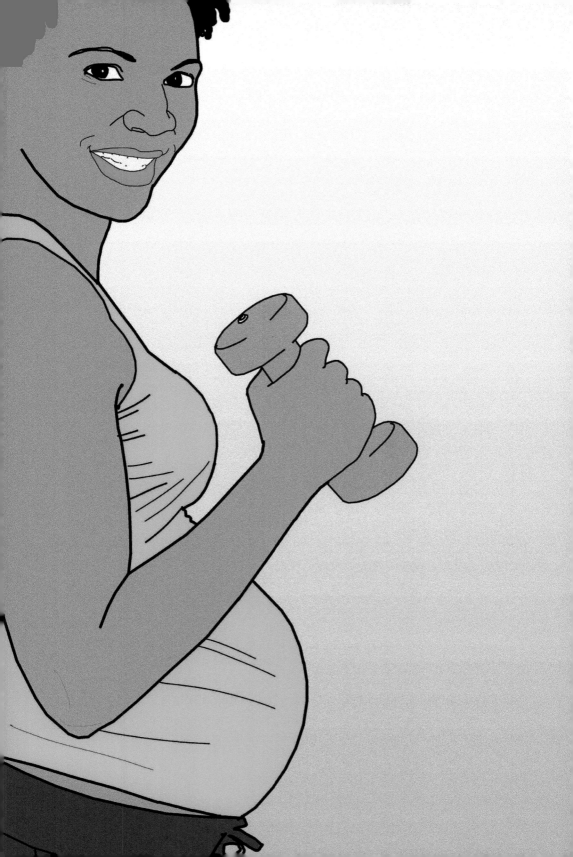

Strengthen your Core: Your central body will start weighing more than the remaining part of your body when you are pregnant. Adopt exercises that strengthen your abdomen and back to have a better balance and posture which will help you cope with the pregnancy related changes.

Exercise Moderately: Anything in excess is bad. For days when I over-pushed myself at the gym, I suffered greatly from it. If you like vigorous and highly intense exercise, it is time to tone down your routine. Too much exercise will only stress out your body. You can choose some more moderate exercises that you can do for a long time.

No Yo-Yo Dieting: Some women might be tempted to get their ideal weight before they put on the extra pounds when pregnant. Are you trying to harm yourself or your baby? Do you even know the content of the concoction you are being given? This is not recommended at all since it might deprive you, and your baby, of the necessary nutrients. Stick to a balanced diet.

Team up with your Partner: We always find only women focusing on their health when trying to conceive, while men do not take care of their fitness. But the truth is your partner's fitness, too, counts in conceiving. Studies have shown that proper exercise can help increase sperm count, so ask your partner to work out with you, it will also increase your time together.

If you are adopting a regimen for yourself, consult your doctor for approval especially if you have some health conditions. He is the best judge of the kind of workout that you might and might not need.

My Experience

As a fitness addict before I got pregnant, it only made more sense for me to continue even while pregnant. I had seen a lot of fit buffs online and read a lot of articles beforehand but the only thing that matters really is YOUR body. While some women go through hell during pregnancy, some are lucky to have it easy. I think I'm in between as I've experienced the good and the bad.

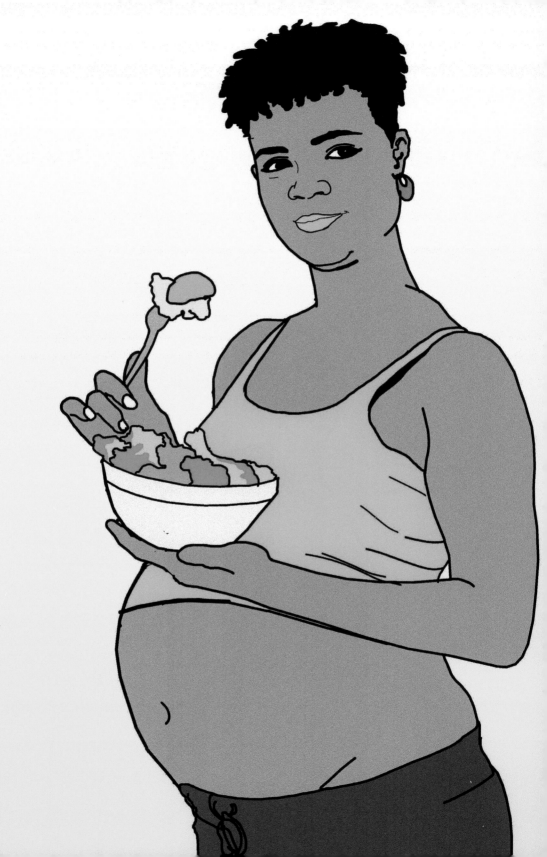

The first trimester went like a breeze and I ran all through. My preggo friend wasn't as fortunate as she was really ill all through the first trimester but I kept encouraging her to eat clean as much as she could. Please note that nutrition is 80% while fitness is 20% and eating a more balanced diet during pregnancy is as good as lifting heavy weights.

During the second trimester, my bump was more visible and I got a bit heavier so I had to slow down my runs from 5miles to 5km and from 4 times a week to 3 times a week. I also reduced my weights before I started

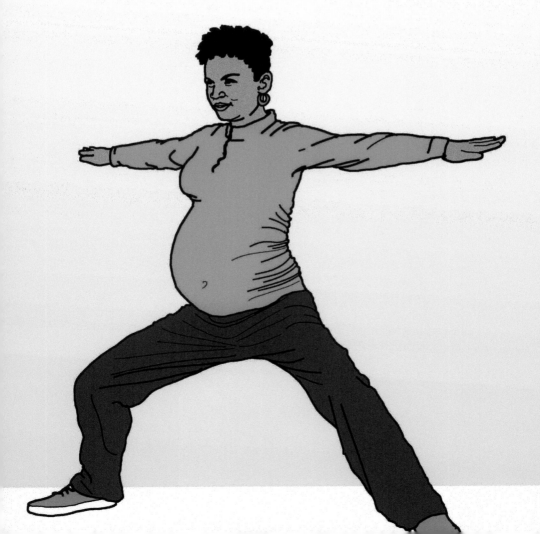

suffering from PPGP (Pregnancy-related Pelvic Girdle Pain) and according to research, this affects one in five women during pregnancy. I was unlucky to be one of the five and the pain was beyond excruciating! I took a break from all hard activities including working out but I introduced Yoga for stretching and I did loads of squats without weights. Even though my midwife said the pain would go on till after delivery, I reminded God of His promises concerning my pregnancy! I woke up one day and the pain was gone! The moment I did not feel pain anymore, I resumed cardio but only in form of brisk walking.

Truth be told, the more active and fit you are during pregnancy, the easier it will be for you to adapt to your shape changing and most importantly your weight gain. I received a lot of positive comments on how I looked during pregnancy but it takes a lot of personal effort.

If you are pregnant and thinking of what exercises to do, I will advise you to continue what you were doing before pregnancy and not introduce your body to new routines. You have to stick to what works for you and not what you see online or at the gym. There are days when I intentionally leave my Oyster card at home so I can enjoy long walks, even though my husband thinks I'm a bit of a weirdo. Lol! If you walk 30 minutes daily throughout your pregnancy, you are better off than someone who sits by the TV all day moaning about being pregnant.

With the amount of energy that comes with the second trimester, it is a good time to put in more work but most importantly, rest when you can! Wear comfortable fitness gears and supportive shoes to keep your balance. Exercise is not dangerous for your baby – there is some evidence that active women are less likely to experience problems in later pregnancy and labour.

I have always wondered what people meant when they say: I'm craving for this or that when pregnant. Are cravings real? Personally, I think it is an illusion. There are days when you feel like eating something even when you are not pregnant, right? Are those cravings for real or people just make up excuses to eat junks? Why are cravings not for vegetables or a glass of water? During my first few weeks of pregnancy, my taste bud became acidic and I wasn't feeling hungry. I realised, I was not interested in the meals I was eating before I got pregnant. I became worried, as this was new to me. What

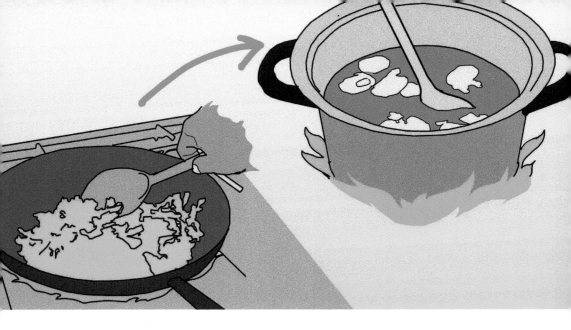

did I do? I swapped all my meals and introduced a new method of cooking them. For instance, instead of making my regular stir-fry, I switched to making soups. Instead of grilling my proteins, I started boiling them, just to have a different flavour. I could not drink milk at all, and I switched to yogurt. I also could not drink water alone; I started cutting in fruits into every glass to aid the desire to quench my thirst.

To be honest, eating well during pregnancy does not necessarily mean eating for two! What if you were expecting a set of quintuplets? Are you going to eat for 6 people? As a woman who is very conscious of what she eats, I had no intentions to gain 100lbs within 9 months! How would I even lose that in a century? Thankfully, having a husband who has been living on a healthy lifestyle also helped greatly.

I monitored my weight gain. I know this may vary amongst women but according to research, you may weigh about 12.5kg (27.6lb) more than you did before you were pregnant. There is absolutely nothing wrong in gaining weight while one is pregnant unless you want your baby to have a stunted growth. It's natural and healthy but don't see this stage as the time to eat all the junks you have been missing out on in life. You'll just be fat beyond recognition and your journey to being a yummy mummy will be a long one! Lol.

I read beforehand on weight expectations, and this is what it looks like, on the average:

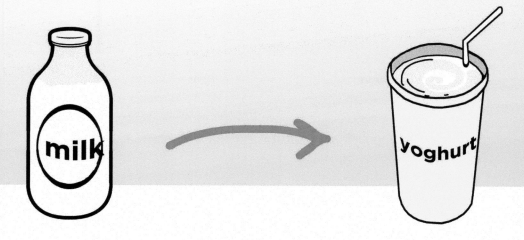

- At birth, a baby weighs about 3.3kg (7.3lb).
- The placenta, which keeps your baby nourished, weighs 0.7kg (1.5lb).
- The amniotic fluid, which supports and cushions your baby, weighs 0.8kg (1.8lb).

The other two thirds of extra weight is due to the changes that happen to your body while you're pregnant. On average:

- The muscle layer of your womb (uterus) grows dramatically, and weighs an extra 0.9kg (2lb).
- Your blood volume increases, and weighs an extra 1.2kg (2.6lb).
- You have extra fluid in your body, weighing about 1.2kg (2.6lb).
- Your breasts weigh an extra 0.4kg (0.9lb).
- You store fat, about 4kg (8.8lb), to give you energy for breastfeeding.

I received loads of compliments on how I looked during my pregnancy but the truth is I took it upon myself to be responsible for my wellbeing during this time. I tracked my weight-gain with the Lifestyle Change with April group and so far I gained 12kg in total and Bryan was 4.5kg at birth.

In the world where people tell you to eat for two, I got very uncomfortable when I tried to overeat. My husband postponed all buffet dates till after delivery as my last experience was not encouraging. Asides my exercise routines, the most important thing to note is being on a healthy weight before getting pregnant and focus on your nutrition during pregnancy. I did not suffer from constipation, diabetes or any health problems. So, how do you achieve a healthy pregnancy weight? It's really not rocket science if you do the following:

1. Stay Healthy: The secret to not being overweight is to stay healthy and be on a healthy weight before getting pregnant. If you are trying to conceive, consider having a change of lifestyle and speak to your GP to figure out if your BMI is on track and how much weight you need to lose.

2. Eat Moderately and Often: I honestly don't know how people starve when trying to lose weight. I plan my day around food and eat the most delicious meals ever. This shouldn't change because you're pregnant and turn you to an unrepentant foodie. You don't need that many extra calories per day to nourish your growing baby. You only need about 340 extra calories per day in your second trimester and 450 extra calories per day in your third trimester IF you are starting pregnancy at a healthy weight. If you're underweight or overweight, these numbers will differ based on your weight gain goal.

3. Cook Your Meals: By making meals at home, you can control the ingredients, and you will wind up with better quality, often for less money. I meal prep every weekend and trust me, not only do I eat what I want when I want to, I also save money! My meals are nutrition packed and less expensive than any takeaway! You can also make your own sweets like quick bread or cookies at home using healthier fats like coconut oil and no sugar.

4. Stay Hydrated: It's important to stay hydrated during pregnancy; I carried my 1litre jar around the house and hit 3 bottles daily. You can do it too, making a big difference in what you drink by staying clear of soda, sweet tea, and sugary fruit drinks and juices! Make your own juices or smoothies, drink some milk for better choices. If you are not in the mood to drink water which is absolutely normal, try some apple juice or orange juice as they are filled with essential vitamins which are important for your baby's development.

5. Snack with Value: My favourite snacks included the following: Fruits (Apples, Grapes, Strawberries, Kiwis, & Bananas) Smoothies, GFK Banana bread, GFK Muffins. Snacking and pregnancy are a good fit: Having smaller, more-frequent snacks helped me ward off morning sickness, indigestion, and heartburn. I loved the way my heart tickled at the sight of yogurt with yummy granola on top! It instantly cures my sweet crunch for anything unhealthy.

6. Indulge: Asides snacking, I will be telling lies if I tell you that I didn't indulge. I did this once a week or once in 2 weeks. My husband always

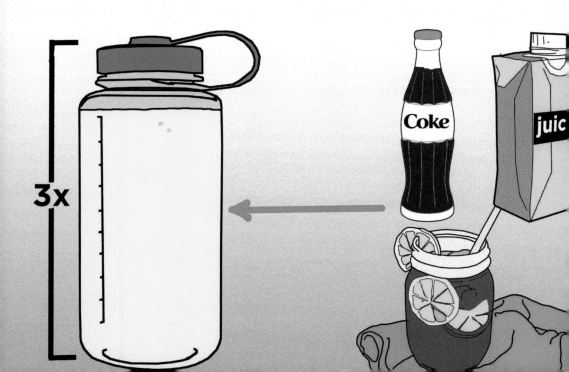

wondered why I kept coins in my wallet all the time. Please o, I didn't deprive myself of a favourite treat at the movies or when I go food shopping. I love ice-cream and burgers and hot chocolates like you do but not daily. We also had our days for take-outs for Chinese, fish and fries, and more.

7. Pick a Routine and Stick to it: Once you have been able to figure out your BMI & nutrition, you need to stay active. Pregnancy gives everyone a very important reason to gain weight and be lazy. Not only was I told that this would ease labour, I also loved the way my arms stayed toned! The simplest workout any pregnant woman can do without costing a penny is walking. 30 minutes daily is better than sitting on your couch or driving. Home workouts are also good, so stop the excuses and stay active with your bump. For every trimester, you will have modified workouts to suit how you feel and how your bump grows.

However, if you are overweight and pregnant, you should not put yourself under any pressure. You should focus on eating healthy and sticking to your meal plan. It will also make so much sense for you not try to go on any funny diet now. Low-calorie or crash diets may make you unwell, and could affect your baby.

I'm keeping my fingers crossed on how much weight you gain overall during your pregnancy and I'm so excited to be part of your journey!

Chapter 12

A Simple Effective Meal Diary

If you bite it, write it.

I f there is anything you want to take seriously on your weight loss journey, it should be keeping a meal diary. The use of a **food diary** can be very effective for keeping your weight goals on target, but many people are hesitant about acting on this idea.

I have been told, it will be "too much work" or "don't know where to get one", or "I am too embarrassed to carry and utilise one in front of others." Excuse me ma, how do you intend to keep track of everything you're putting in your mouth? If you bite it, write it!

If your goal is to eat 1,500 calories a day, having a journal to document all that you are eating puts things in perspective for you. It helps you pinpoint your protein intake, if you are eating enough vegetables, if you are eating whole grains more than white flour, and eating whole fruits. It helps you find places where you can reduce calories that add to your bottom line (literally), such as mindless drinks, eating off your kid's plate, or how many vending machine snacks you eat in a week, just for example.

It can also help you monitor your successes in your food plan. It shows if you tried quinoa, kale or goat meat for the first time. You will know if you are drinking enough water to stay properly hydrated for your exercise output. You can then evaluate if you are feeling more energetic. A food diary is a great tool that helps **ONLY YOU**! You can find digital varieties online but this will come in handy for you.

How do you set about keeping a food diary?

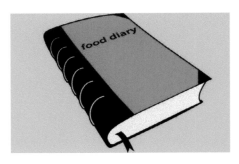

You can start a food journal without any professional help at all. The only thing you need is a little of your time and dedication. You will have to be consistent in putting down everything that goes into your mouth. Do not skip registering meals, and keep track of even the smallest snacks that you chew mindlessly while watching a movie. Those extra peanuts? Write them down! If writing everything down meticulously is really problematic, make use of this chapter to make the job of registering different meals in different parts of town much easier.

How to keep food log in the most effective way

Think about it this way. Remember when you first had a love diary and you wrote everything about that first kiss? ☺ Remember how you guarded the diary so jealously because of the honesty of the content. Be that honest with this and take heed of these simple tips to make your food diary the great help it can be.

- First, consider the format. You will certainly need to register how hungry you felt as you sat down to eat, when you had your meal, what did you take and what amount?
- You may encounter certain difficulties, be ready to cope with them.
- In case you find it hard holding yourself in check, make a point of measuring out and weighing all your food.
- If calories are the big problem, **check the calorie content of every food item before you buy it.** Pay attention to serving sizes. If a nutritional label says the entire package has about 4 servings, then divide the entire contents of the package into 4 even groups. One group is equal to one serving.
- For a clearer picture of your eating habits, include the information on where you take your meals, with whom, and whether there were any additional circumstances.
- If eating is linked with emotional issues, register your moods both before and after the meal (or the snack).
- Practically speaking, this journal should be kept on a daily basis, but if you find it inconvenient for some reason or other, make a decision to fill it at least five days every week.
- Expect it to get easier.

Decide how you are going to keep your food log: either fill it out after each meal or find some time every evening to concentrate on what you had.

Decide what information you will really need

The idea that your food diary should contain full details, otherwise it will be useless, is wrong. Just start recording information, and soon your food log will be helping you analyse and understand your eating habits like you have never done before.

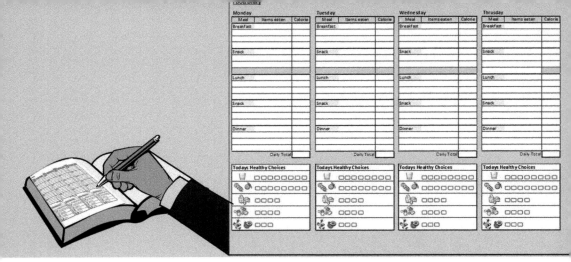

Add up every little bit

As you become more accurate, writing all those pinches of fries, handfuls of sweets from the office, random sauces and mayonnaise that went with your snacks, you will be able to trace those unwanted calories that keep you stagnant. Reading your food journal backwards, you will see the way all those small items add up and amount to many more calories.

Look up calories on nutritional websites.

Not all foods have packaging that shows the number of calories, but there are many websites that tell you the calories of nearly any food. Just make sure that after you check the calories for a 4-oz. piece of fish, for example, you eat only that much.

Register portion sizes

Make the picture of your meals more precise by jotting down exact portion sizes for every dish in your diary. Especially when you are away from home, while you measure out the portions, you will gain a better understanding of what is a normal portion for you. Once you have gotten the knack of it, you will remember your portions and do it later on a less regular basis.

Consider the problems that will be facing you

You may be embarrassed about your eating habits and you do not want to keep them registered. You believe that keeping a food log is an absolutely worthless suggestion that will not lead to any progress. It may be extremely inconvenient for you to keep detailed accounts after each meal with your lifestyle. When you indulge, you feel so bad that you want to give it up. All, or some, of these considerations are sure to occur to you at one time or another. Yet all of them are not as drastic as they may seem. Keep your mind on the usefulness of the food log, leave down the slips on the way, do not try to be perfect and focus on controlling your habits.

Once you have got a well-filled diary, read it from the beginning and you will realise the full use of it. After doing it on your own, send your diary to an expert like April or a therapist and go over it with them: they can point out the things you missed or suggest ways to alter your eating habits. The more you analyse the information, the more benefits you will draw from it.

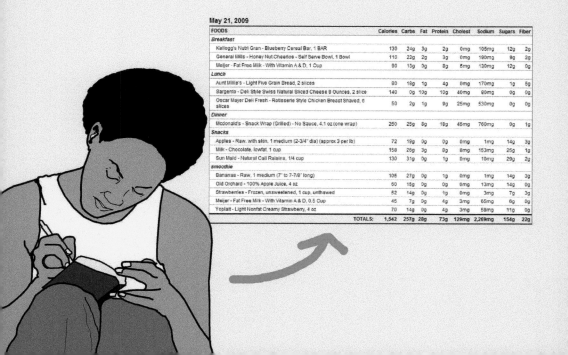

May 21, 2009

FOODS	Calories	Carbs	Fat	Protein	Cholest	Sodium	Sugars	Fiber
Breakfast								
Kellogg's Nutri Grain - Blueberry Cereal Bar, 1 BAR	130	24g	3g	2g	0mg	105mg	12g	2g
General Mills - Honey Nut Cheerios - Self Serve Bowl, 1 Bowl	110	22g	2g	3g	0mg	190mg	9g	2g
Meijer - Fat Free Milk - With Vitamin A & D, 1 Cup	90	13g	0g	8g	5mg	130mg	12g	0g
Lunch								
Aunt Millie's - Light Five Grain Bread, 2 slices	80	18g	1g	4g	0mg	170mg	1g	5g
Sargento - Deli Style Swiss Natural Sliced Cheese 8 Ounces, 2 slice	140	0g	10g	10g	40mg	80mg	0g	0g
Oscar Mayer Deli Fresh - Rotisserie Style Chicken Breast Shaved, 6 slices	50	2g	1g	9g	25mg	530mg	0g	0g
Dinner								
Mcdonald's - Snack Wrap (Grilled) - No Sauce, 4.1 oz (one wrap)	250	25g	8g	18g	45mg	760mg	0g	1g
Snacks								
Apples - Raw, with skin, 1 medium (2-3/4" dia) (approx 3 per lb)	72	19g	0g	0g	0mg	1mg	14g	3g
Milk - Chocolate, lowfat, 1 cup	158	26g	3g	8g	8mg	153mg	25g	1g
Sun Maid - Natural Cali Raisins, 1/4 cup	130	31g	0g	1g	0mg	10mg	29g	2g
smoothie								
Bananas - Raw, 1 medium (7" to 7-7/8" long)	105	27g	0g	1g	0mg	1mg	14g	3g
Old Orchard - 100% Apple Juice, 4 oz	60	15g	0g	0g	0mg	13mg	14g	0g
Strawberries - Frozen, unsweetened, 1 cup, unthawed	52	14g	0g	1g	0mg	3mg	7g	3g
Meijer - Fat Free Milk - With Vitamin A & D, 0.5 Cup	45	7g	0g	4g	3mg	65mg	6g	0g
Yoplait - Light Nonfat Creamy Strawberry, 4 oz	70	14g	0g	4g	3mg	58mg	11g	0g
TOTALS:	**1,542**	**257g**	**28g**	**73g**	**129mg**	**2,269mg**	**154g**	**22g**

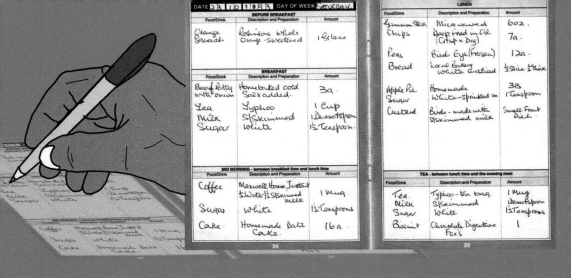

Whatever your goal is, you can achieve it. Is it to keep calorie count? To drop a dress size or to balance out your eating? A food journal will provide you with a scientific, holistic means of achieving them. You will hone your awareness, discover recurring patterns, make your bad habits stand out and consequently make necessary alterations more obvious. A little commitment and a few minutes of your time will go a long way.

Let's get writing! You can print out this page for as many copies you will need.

		Meal	Calories	Water	Additional Comments
Monday	Breakfast				
	Lunch				
	Dinner				
	Snacks				
		Meal	Calories	Water	Additional Comments
Tuesday	Breakfast				
	Lunch				
	Dinner				
	Snacks				
		Meal	Calories	Water	Additional Comments
Wednesday	Breakfast				
	Lunch				
	Dinner				
	Snacks				
		Meal	Calories	Water	Additional Comments
Thursday	Breakfast				
	Lunch				
	Dinner				
	Snacks				
		Meal	Calories	Water	Additional Comments
Friday	Breakfast				
	Lunch				
	Dinner				
	Snacks				
		Meal	Calories	Water	Additional Comments
Saturday	Breakfast				
	Lunch				
	Dinner				
	Snacks				
		Meal	Calories	Water	Additional Comments
Sunday	Breakfast				
	Lunch				
	Dinner				
	Snacks				

		Meal	Calories	Water	Additional Comments
Monday	Breakfast				
	Lunch				
	Dinner				
	Snacks				

		Meal	Calories	Water	Additional Comments
Tuesday	Breakfast				
	Lunch				
	Dinner				
	Snacks				

		Meal	Calories	Water	Additional Comments
Wednesday	Breakfast				
	Lunch				
	Dinner				
	Snacks				

		Meal	Calories	Water	Additional Comments
Thursday	Breakfast				
	Lunch				
	Dinner				
	Snacks				

		Meal	Calories	Water	Additional Comments
Friday	Breakfast				
	Lunch				
	Dinner				
	Snacks				

		Meal	Calories	Water	Additional Comments
Saturday	Breakfast				
	Lunch				
	Dinner				
	Snacks				

		Meal	Calories	Water	Additional Comments
Sunday	Breakfast				
	Lunch				
	Dinner				
	Snacks				

		Meal	Calories	Water	Additional Comments
Monday	Breakfast				
	Lunch				
	Dinner				
	Snacks				

		Meal	Calories	Water	Additional Comments
Tuesday	Breakfast				
	Lunch				
	Dinner				
	Snacks				

		Meal	Calories	Water	Additional Comments
Wednesday	Breakfast				
	Lunch				
	Dinner				
	Snacks				

		Meal	Calories	Water	Additional Comments
Thursday	Breakfast				
	Lunch				
	Dinner				
	Snacks				

		Meal	Calories	Water	Additional Comments
Friday	Breakfast				
	Lunch				
	Dinner				
	Snacks				

		Meal	Calories	Water	Additional Comments
Saturday	Breakfast				
	Lunch				
	Dinner				
	Snacks				

		Meal	Calories	Water	Additional Comments
Sunday	Breakfast				
	Lunch				
	Dinner				
	Snacks				

	Meal	Calories	Water	Additional Comments
Monday Breakfast				
Lunch				
Dinner				
Snacks				

	Meal	Calories	Water	Additional Comments
Tuesday Breakfast				
Lunch				
Dinner				
Snacks				

	Meal	Calories	Water	Additional Comments
Wednesday Breakfast				
Lunch				
Dinner				
Snacks				

	Meal	Calories	Water	Additional Comments
Thursday Breakfast				
Lunch				
Dinner				
Snacks				

	Meal	Calories	Water	Additional Comments
Friday Breakfast				
Lunch				
Dinner				
Snacks				

	Meal	Calories	Water	Additional Comments
Saturday Breakfast				
Lunch				
Dinner				
Snacks				

	Meal	Calories	Water	Additional Comments
Sunday Breakfast				
Lunch				
Dinner				
Snacks				

	Meal	Calories	Water	Additional Comments
Monday				
Breakfast				
Lunch				
Dinner				
Snacks				

	Meal	Calories	Water	Additional Comments
Tuesday				
Breakfast				
Lunch				
Dinner				
Snacks				

	Meal	Calories	Water	Additional Comments
Wednesday				
Breakfast				
Lunch				
Dinner				
Snacks				

	Meal	Calories	Water	Additional Comments
Thursday				
Breakfast				
Lunch				
Dinner				
Snacks				

	Meal	Calories	Water	Additional Comments
Friday				
Breakfast				
Lunch				
Dinner				
Snacks				

	Meal	Calories	Water	Additional Comments
Saturday				
Breakfast				
Lunch				
Dinner				
Snacks				

	Meal	Calories	Water	Additional Comments
Sunday				
Breakfast				
Lunch				
Dinner				
Snacks				

		Meal	Calories	Water	Additional Comments
Monday	Breakfast				
	Lunch				
	Dinner				
	Snacks				

		Meal	Calories	Water	Additional Comments
Tuesday	Breakfast				
	Lunch				
	Dinner				
	Snacks				

		Meal	Calories	Water	Additional Comments
Wednesday	Breakfast				
	Lunch				
	Dinner				
	Snacks				

		Meal	Calories	Water	Additional Comments
Thursday	Breakfast				
	Lunch				
	Dinner				
	Snacks				

		Meal	Calories	Water	Additional Comments
Friday	Breakfast				
	Lunch				
	Dinner				
	Snacks				

		Meal	Calories	Water	Additional Comments
Saturday	Breakfast				
	Lunch				
	Dinner				
	Snacks				

		Meal	Calories	Water	Additional Comments
Sunday	Breakfast				
	Lunch				
	Dinner				
	Snacks				

		Meal	Calories	Water	Additional Comments
Monday	Breakfast				
	Lunch				
	Dinner				
	Snacks				
Tuesday	Breakfast				
	Lunch				
	Dinner				
	Snacks				
Wednesday	Breakfast				
	Lunch				
	Dinner				
	Snacks				
Thursday	Breakfast				
	Lunch				
	Dinner				
	Snacks				
Friday	Breakfast				
	Lunch				
	Dinner				
	Snacks				
Saturday	Breakfast				
	Lunch				
	Dinner				
	Snacks				
Sunday	Breakfast				
	Lunch				
	Dinner				
	Snacks				

	Meal	Calories	Water	Additional Comments
Monday	Breakfast			
	Lunch			
	Dinner			
	Snacks			

	Meal	Calories	Water	Additional Comments
Tuesday	Breakfast			
	Lunch			
	Dinner			
	Snacks			

	Meal	Calories	Water	Additional Comments
Wednesday	Breakfast			
	Lunch			
	Dinner			
	Snacks			

	Meal	Calories	Water	Additional Comments
Thursday	Breakfast			
	Lunch			
	Dinner			
	Snacks			

	Meal	Calories	Water	Additional Comments
Friday	Breakfast			
	Lunch			
	Dinner			
	Snacks			

	Meal	Calories	Water	Additional Comments
Saturday	Breakfast			
	Lunch			
	Dinner			
	Snacks			

	Meal	Calories	Water	Additional Comments
Sunday	Breakfast			
	Lunch			
	Dinner			
	Snacks			

	Meal	Calories	Water	Additional Comments
Monday	Breakfast			
	Lunch			
	Dinner			
	Snacks			

	Meal	Calories	Water	Additional Comments
Tuesday	Breakfast			
	Lunch			
	Dinner			
	Snacks			

	Meal	Calories	Water	Additional Comments
Wednesday	Breakfast			
	Lunch			
	Dinner			
	Snacks			

	Meal	Calories	Water	Additional Comments
Thursday	Breakfast			
	Lunch			
	Dinner			
	Snacks			

	Meal	Calories	Water	Additional Comments
Friday	Breakfast			
	Lunch			
	Dinner			
	Snacks			

	Meal	Calories	Water	Additional Comments
Saturday	Breakfast			
	Lunch			
	Dinner			
	Snacks			

	Meal	Calories	Water	Additional Comments
Sunday	Breakfast			
	Lunch			
	Dinner			
	Snacks			

		Meal	Calories	Water	Additional Comments
Monday	Breakfast				
	Lunch				
	Dinner				
	Snacks				

		Meal	Calories	Water	Additional Comments
Tuesday	Breakfast				
	Lunch				
	Dinner				
	Snacks				

		Meal	Calories	Water	Additional Comments
Wednesday	Breakfast				
	Lunch				
	Dinner				
	Snacks				

		Meal	Calories	Water	Additional Comments
Thursday	Breakfast				
	Lunch				
	Dinner				
	Snacks				

		Meal	Calories	Water	Additional Comments
Friday	Breakfast				
	Lunch				
	Dinner				
	Snacks				

		Meal	Calories	Water	Additional Comments
Saturday	Breakfast				
	Lunch				
	Dinner				
	Snacks				

		Meal	Calories	Water	Additional Comments
Sunday	Breakfast				
	Lunch				
	Dinner				
	Snacks				

		Meal	Calories	Water	Additional Comments
Monday	Breakfast				
	Lunch				
	Dinner				
	Snacks				
		Meal	Calories	Water	Additional Comments
Tuesday	Breakfast				
	Lunch				
	Dinner				
	Snacks				
		Meal	Calories	Water	Additional Comments
Wednesday	Breakfast				
	Lunch				
	Dinner				
	Snacks				
		Meal	Calories	Water	Additional Comments
Thursday	Breakfast				
	Lunch				
	Dinner				
	Snacks				
		Meal	Calories	Water	Additional Comments
Friday	Breakfast				
	Lunch				
	Dinner				
	Snacks				
		Meal	Calories	Water	Additional Comments
Saturday	Breakfast				
	Lunch				
	Dinner				
	Snacks				
		Meal	Calories	Water	Additional Comments
Sunday	Breakfast				
	Lunch				
	Dinner				
	Snacks				

	Meal	Calories	Water	Additional Comments
Monday	Breakfast			
	Lunch			
	Dinner			
	Snacks			

	Meal	Calories	Water	Additional Comments
Tuesday	Breakfast			
	Lunch			
	Dinner			
	Snacks			

	Meal	Calories	Water	Additional Comments
Wednesday	Breakfast			
	Lunch			
	Dinner			
	Snacks			

	Meal	Calories	Water	Additional Comments
Thursday	Breakfast			
	Lunch			
	Dinner			
	Snacks			

	Meal	Calories	Water	Additional Comments
Friday	Breakfast			
	Lunch			
	Dinner			
	Snacks			

	Meal	Calories	Water	Additional Comments
Saturday	Breakfast			
	Lunch			
	Dinner			
	Snacks			

	Meal	Calories	Water	Additional Comments
Sunday	Breakfast			
	Lunch			
	Dinner			
	Snacks			

Chapter 13

Dear April...

In this chapter, you will learn about different women's journeys on the #LifestylechangewithApril road. Different women are on a journey for different purposes. Many of them I have never met. Read. Enjoy. Get motivated. Start your own journey.

How do I start? Ok, I heard about April Laugh through Instagram at the beginning of the year. I was scrolling through the newsfeed one afternoon when I came across a friend's picture, which was @ Fitmrsfats. So I followed on to see, which I usually do, then I saw all these amazing pictures of women—and one man— who has lost weight there. I saw Genevieve, my secondary school friend, with these beautiful pictures on Facebook. I was wondering how this was achieved because it did not seem real to me. So I started following @ Fitmrsfats and then, the stalking started.

Fast forward to March, I mustered the courage to contact Lola via email. She replied quickly with the pricing for the 12-week plan. The price, by the way, was too good to be true. I pleaded with her to keep a place for me in April till I get the money as there were few spaces left. God so good, I got to join the April cohort 2017.

When I got the meal plan, I was confused. There were no pills or shakes to it—a previous personal trainer had me on shakes and pills for 4months. Interesting! Seeing food, I was happy because I love food; my problem was the exercises, but the ladies I met in the group were on fire. They really meant business; they kept going and this made me go for more. This is the best decision I have made in my life so far. The results are outstanding; I could not believe it. I am here now and looking at myself and thinking: is this really me? God is good; some people think I have had a gastric band to help me lose weight and I keep telling them, April has my back. I am over the moon with my results even though I've not hit my target; I am more than happy with the results. Recommendation yes, and can't wait for them to contact Lola. Thank you so much, I owe you all a lot; this new Nana is all down to every one of you. Please everyone stop sleeping o, and start working for your new body because with April, you get 200 out of 100.

Love you Queens,
Nana

Nana

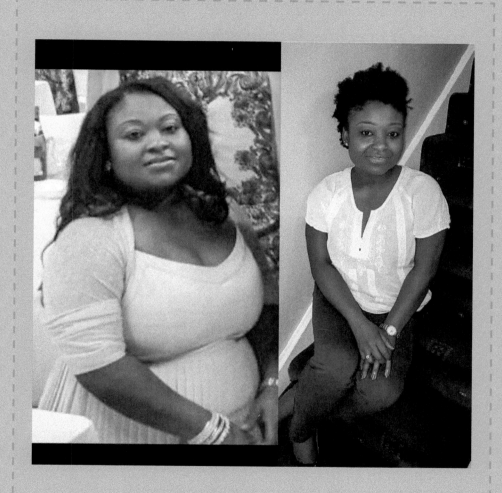

Genevieve

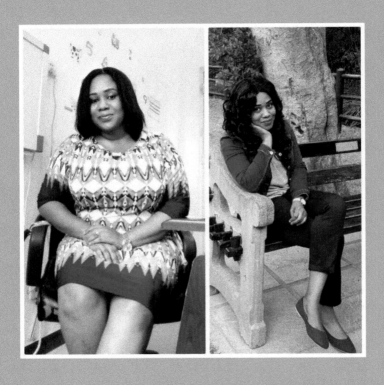

For over a decade, I saw the weight creeping up on me and I could not do anything about it. I hated it, but I did not even know where to start. Fast forward to October 2016, weighing a whopping 105kgs, with high blood pressure, no self-confidence and feeling miserable about my body, while I was browsing Instagram, I came across @fitmrsfats and saw some amazing transformations! I was impressed but I still did not believe I could do it. One fine afternoon, while eating ice cream and cake in bed after work, I sent her an email. She got back to me and gave me all the details. I threw caution to the wind and signed up with her. When she got my body statistics and told me I had to lose 33kgs, I almost told her that would not be possible; so I was no longer interested. So, I encouraged myself and told myself to take it a day at a time. She made me write down my goals, and I said I wanted to lose the 33kgs in 12 months. So we started! After two weeks, I had lost 4.8kg! That was when I knew I was in the right place! Six and a half months later, I lost the weight and was at my ideal healthy weight! To say I feel good is an understatement. I feel awesome. I feel strong. My blood pressure has normalised. I'm in a better place. Believe me, if I can do it, you can do it too! It takes a lot of discipline and dedication, but it is doable. The people doing it don't have two heads or four legs! In as much as we invest in clothes, shoes, and expensive wigs, we must invest in our health too! Thank you very much April @fitmrsfats and all the amazing ladies on this journey! We did this together!

--Genevieve

"So, I decided to do something about my weight; eating habits and fitness level. My first workout, as part of the group, was on 23rd of May, 2016. It is one year today that I signed up to ALF group; have I reached my desired weight? NO, (food won't let somebody be great!) but I have gained so much more in the past year—no, not the weight. Let me share some of my new knowledge with you.

Fitness and healthy eating

A year ago, if someone told me I could run half a marathon in 1.27hrs in my living room, I would have said in another lifetime. If someone had said that I could go a whole week without eating RICE? I would have said they were joking. Guess what? I actually didn't eat rice for a month!

Endurance

I have learnt to push myself beyond my comfort zone, and do things that I never imagined I could do, like go running at 4.30am after only 2 hours of sleep!

Spiritual Growth

I have seen a change in this area of my life, as my running time doubles up as my prayer, worship and soul searching time. I also challenged myself this year to pray or study the bible for the same length of time I work out, which is a minimum of 30minutes; this is still work in progress.

Relationships / Sisterhood

Where do I start from? Okay, I never knew it was possible to form close/tight/strong bonds with people I have never set eyes on, in different time zones and different parts of the world. This is what I have gained most from joining this group, and it is also very precious to me.

- *There are ladies that have left the group and I still chat with them on a regular basis*
- *There is a particular lady who I call my lover; I chat with her more than I do my husband! My husband has adopted her as his sister; we even have a WhatsApp group for the three of us and we have never met her.*
- *I never knew it was possible to meet and know someone for less than a year who loves your children like they are hers, and your children prefer to stay in her house rather than come home!*
- *When a lady you've never met and lives in a different country from you decides to adopt your daughter as her own, and decides to make you the voice of reason with regards to issues she's dealing with!*
- *Ladies that would ask you to join and agree with them in prayer on issues pertaining to their family, marriage, and more. I could go on and on but it just amazes me at the bonds I have formed in the past year. I also have more connections or reach in Nigeria, Norway, USA and Australia.*

Instagram posts

It is humbling when people say they get inspired from my IG post to start working out, and some of them even signed up to the group. One of the kids I used to look after in church who is now in his early 20s actually said to me, "Aunty, it's good to see people of your age group working out, please keep it up!"

I really thank God for April, it was a video of her on IG working out while pregnant that pushed me to do something about my lifestyle, rather than just keep moaning and do nothing! My relationship with her has gone beyond a lifestyle change coach, and I now consider her a sister. That's my year in a nutshell"

--Toyin Kayode

Being small in size takes me back to many years ago that I can't even remember. I have always struggled with my weight; thanks to EXTREMELY bad eating habits and laziness. I once gave this weight loss / detox a try back in 2007-2008 with the terrible Beyonce Maple Syrup diet which led me to drop a few pounds, but that didn't last very long as the weight crept back on me and took me to even bigger sizes.

In 2012, I then came across the Cambridge Diet. I met up with the Cambridge Weight Loss consultant; she explained the diet to me and started me with the strictest diet. I was required to attend weigh-in sessions every week. The first week of exclusively just drinking these terrible shakes, I lost about 8 pounds. At this stage, I was encouraged to continue, not knowing this was a very unhealthy way of losing the weight. Whilst I was on the programme, I lost about 4 stones but had to stop as I was losing quite a lot of money on a weekly basis. I was spending an average of £45-£50 per week on these shakes at the time, and did it for about four months. The main reason I put a stop to this diet was because I ended up at the hospital with terrible stomach cramps, and the doctors were telling me I was developing gallstones. At this stage, I decided to quit, although the consultant advised that the Cambridge had nothing to do with it. I spoke with my GP and asked for a referral to the gym. They did the referral. I joined but wasn't active; I found every excuse not to go and still eat the same food I would normally eat.

I gained all the weight back, lost all my confidence, tried doing the weight loss on my own and all, with no success. Then I came across the ABLE FITMRSFATS as my very good friend and sister, has enrolled into her programme and the difference in the before and after pictures spoke VOLUME. My friend took so much time to explain how the plan worked and said many good things about April. After discussions with my husband, I promised myself this would be my last bus-stop. It all started from an email to April. From her prompt response to her constant support and availability, it has been an amazing journey so far. I was excited when I saw the meal plan she provided. I was like 'ehn, so I can eat Naija food and lose the weight! Oya, let's go there!' So, I started embracing the meal prepping and this definitely kept me on track. I had all the equipment I required to embark on this journey, apart from my watch, and just immediately got straight into it. The first weigh-in, I was quite nervous as I hadn't stepped on the scale for two weeks, and was really excited to see the weight drop by 4.5kg by just eating right, exercising and drinking water.

The experience has been totally amazing, and I know there is no looking back from here. I am far from where I need to be but I am confident I will get there as I take each day at a time. April has made me realise that I can put my mind to do whatever I want to accomplish. It would be very unfair to not give credit to whom credit is due. The ladies in the group are just beyond AMAZING! The support is seriously out of this world; I have never seen such in my life.

April and my lovely ladies, you guys rock! I look forward to the rest of this journey with every one of you. I am nowhere near where I need to be, but I am glad I am not where I used to be. My energies are right up there; I enjoy working out and carrying out my own research on foods and the effects they have on your body."

--Bola

Dearest April Laugh,

Knowing you has been such a pleasure. At home, April Laugh comes up in our conversations so often. You have become family. For years, I tried to control my slow and creeping weight gain. I ran for two years with local runners. I drank green tea and other drinks. I ate lean. I ate mean. I tried this diet and that diet. I rode a bicycle but decided I did not want to die by HCGs. I learnt to swim for a year, but my hair suffered loss. The weight just kept coming. I decided I was not going to size 13 as size 12 was becoming tight! I used a waist band but decided there was more to life than this! They all gave a temporary solution. There had to be a more realistic one.

I found you because I was angry. I heard a Nigerian lady had dumped Nigerian meals in order to diet successfully. I decided only Nigerians can promote Nigeria. I googled 'dieting on Nigerian food' and found you! I followed you for a while on Instagram and then, also went back in time to EVERY Instagram post of yours. I read others too, but decided to go with you.

This has indeed been a lifestyle change. I loved your lack of trust in others; you needed evidence! Welcome to my turf. You needed people with motivation, I lacked none. What a lifestyle change! I never drank so much water in my life, or ate so much vegetable. You call it eating clean. I began to use your language too; "what a wow!"

And slowly, the weight dropped. And the comments followed. Six weeks later, I got my first comment: "whatever you are doing, it is working!" The lady that sits behind me in church said I changed right before her eyes! A lady in bible school almost screamed and said, "you have lost so much weight!" A third lady said she needed to join me and so, I introduced her to you. Finally, my pastor's wife said to me, "I do have to go the gym Simi, don't I?"

My husband is leaner; he was never fat. He is tall, dark and handsome but with a lil tummy but boy, have things changed? This year has indeed been 'EPIC' and I am so blessed to have you. My favourite quote from you is "shut up and run!" I wish I could say it out loud, but since you don't, then I won't. Thank you APRIL LAUGH.

-Dr Sinmi Ajike

Where do I start? It has been a great journey. I signed up for the "Lifestyle Change with April" on a whim. A few months before, I had checked out the website and let it go but I kept thinking about it because I knew I had to do something about my weight. With menopause here and an empty nest creeping up on me, I needed to get a grip. The accountability is what has helped me greatly. I have lost count of the number of times I negotiated with myself in the morning about my workouts or on Sundays, about my meal prep! I knew I had to do it. I'm not quite near my goal yet, but now, I know it is possible. The one thing I am thankful for is what I have learnt about myself: I can do anything if I put my mind to it. I cannot end this without saying anything about April (Auntie March): the queen bee herself! She is a motivator; she is not playing! When you think you have not got it in you, she helps you find it to continue. The hive is so supportive. We take care of each other and given that we live miles apart and only met on the platform, that is awesome. Thank you April and thank you to the ladies. Bless! Bless! Bless!

--Akwelley

Coach!! I was at the tailor's just this past weekend. I have been using her for a long time so I know her measurements are always perfect! I mean, no need for adjustments when I go for fittings, ever! She had my measurements taken a month ago, as soon as I tried the dress on, she said: "Kofo, you must have lost weight." It's so obvious I couldn't deny it as the dress looked like a sack of rice on me, and she was moaning about how I'm giving her double job *side eye* Hey! Girl is looking fly, double job or not!

My mom also saw me and said, in Yoruba, "this thing you are doing, you should stop. Your neck is now long." Asides countless compliments from family and friends, I feel confident and good within, and can now wear some clothes I already thought would be given out because they couldn't fit few months ago. Never thought it would be easy when I was about to sign up because I was breastfeeding, and I obviously love my food. After procrastinating several times, I signed up and it's amazing how April's plan is to EAT and still lose weight ☺ Each prep day, my husband would say: "with all these 'orisirisi' you are cooking, are you sure you are on a diet?"

Thank you so much for not being selfish. Thank you for choosing to share your knowledge with us. My weight this morning was 68.7 (from 78). I am not where I want to be, but will continue to keep the flag up and make you proud. God bless you and your family, your coast will be enlarged mightily.

--Kofo

If you told me eight weeks ago, that I would look like this a few weeks down the line, I would have denied it. It can only be God who brought me to your page' April Laugh Fitness; I got in touch with April as I had been following the page quietly. We spoke and again, I put it on the side for another year. *laughing out loud* Procrastination is the devil. Then this year, I got the courage to go for it after years of excuses upon excuses. After ten years of carrying this extra fat, I ended up just dressing in baggy tops and jeans, never fitted dresses. I carried this well as I have never been too big, but the struggle was the bulging tummy area and big arms. April Laugh is the best. I've always known what to do in terms of eating healthy and exercising because of my line of work, but I needed discipline, accountability and motivation. That's exactly what I needed from the fitfam group of ladies! We eat very well and exercise, and that's what I enjoy on this journey. I feel so energetic and revived, and my kids have even noticed the difference, even my soon-to-be 18-year-old! Not only am I on a journey to lose weight, but to a healthier me! I'm not at the finishing line yet, but I am definitely getting there. Anyway, there is no finishing line, it is a lifestyle change and I'm loving it! Thank you so much Coach and Fithive family!

--Sue

It is twelve weeks already? Where did the time go? I am definitely loving the new me. I am not where I want to be yet, but not where I used to be. I got to meet this amazing Mrs Fats through my sister-in-love, Dr Temz. I woke up to her transformation pictures a couple of months ago, and I was like "WOW." I just kept bombarding her with questions like how did you do it? What happened to you? It was just like magic to be. You see, the Temi I know is a lover of good and unhealthy food, just like me. I also know she has a crazy schedule, just like me as well. So, I was just wondering how was she able to do this? So, she gave me coach's email. I didn't even wait till the next day; I sent that email on the spot. My life has never been the same since then.

My food choices have changed. My exercise has been regular. Thanks to my monitoring spirit coach. Guys, she's got a monitoring spirit o, like I get scared to cheat even though she's thousands of miles away, it's always as if she's right in front of me whispering: if you dare!

Thanks to my amazing Fithive sisters for the daily motivation.

--Labake

"I woke up one day and just hated how I looked! I had spent the last four to five years making excuses while the weight piled up. I was honestly trying to lose weight but I guess I wasn't doing the right things. October, 2016, I decided I was tired of hating my body. I found @fitmrsfats, who is not just a coach, but my sister now. She whipped me into shape, literally! No excuses allowed!

The rest is history. 20+ kilos down, everyone is begging me to stop. I'm loving my body. I love my new lifestyle. My health is so much better. I just realised I haven't taken most of my meds in the last two months, and my energy level is off the charts...and of course, my confidence has taken a boost! I sure love the new me.

--Temi

Temi

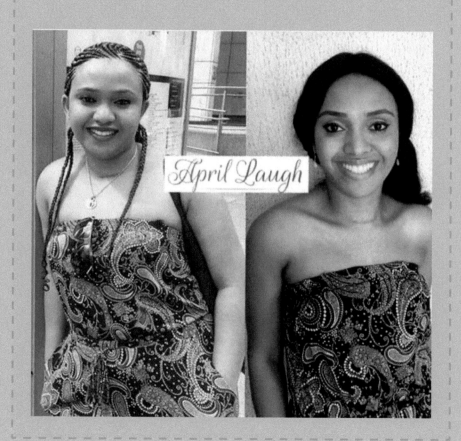

When I first met April, I was taken aback. She was so friendly, sounded like she'd known me for years. *laughs out loud* Usually, Nigerian women aren't like that – you know yourself! However, when she started to ask me questions about my goals, my challenges and then, told me we had work to do, I knew she meant business-very professional, 100 per cent, eyes on the ball! I started gradually, setting my personal goals. My workout sessions started in a week but couldn't burn so much calories. Gradually, I increased the calorie burn as my stamina improved and now, I can work out for an hour continuously. What a WoW!

Food prep was a challenge too but when I struggled, I called coach and by the time I finished talking to her, I understood the problem and the solution. The motivation on the group is amazing. These women are mothers, professionals and entrepreneurs, and still had time to make everyday count! So, I knew I had to up my game; no excuses. On days I felt I wanted to take a break, someone will post their sweatfie, transformation picture, and that will be the end of the idea of a break *laughing out loud*

What I have discovered about myself so far is that I have tenacity, and it's being transferred to other areas of my life, and I have dear Lola to thank for it. It's truly a lifestyle change journey. The journey continues.

--Abi

Abi

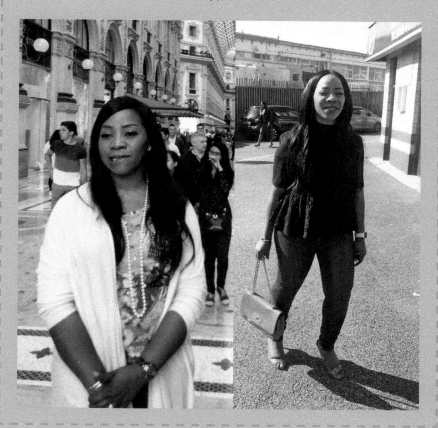

Keeping fit and staying healthy is one of the personal goals I set some months ago after my milestone birthday. I can't remember how I dabbled on April Laugh's page on IG; the results were beyond my belief so I decided to contact her. It's been a life changing experience; I feel great and energetic all the time. My fitness and endurance has improved tremendously, from brisk-walking to running half-marathon without stopping. I'm more knowledgeable about healthy food choices and lifestyle.

--Lola

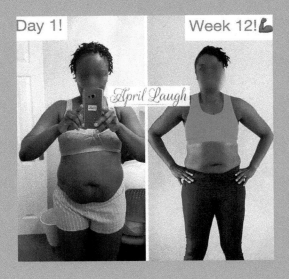

Wow! What a journey it's been so far, and we're not even done yet! Following a recommendation from my friend, Kemi, I joined April Laugh's FitFam around the same time I moved to a new country to start a new job. At the time, I knew I was already overweight for my frame, and was concerned about how it would deteriorate with the travelling lifestyle of my new job. I knew it was time to make radical change and Lola's magic formula was what I needed. I've truly seen a change in my mentality towards food; I am happily making better choices and working out. I can barely believe that I run now—I've always hated running. Dare I say that; I'm enjoying it! I'm not yet at my target weight, but I'm pretty excited about the progress we've made so far! Yes, 'we' – Lola and my motivational sisters in the FitFam. Lola, may God continue to bless you and expand your empire!

PS: There's no magic! It's simply a lifestyle change and I'm bikini ready!
--Timi

My struggle has always been with accountability. I've always known how to work out and eat right but for some reason, I'm entirely dependent on a support system for encouragement. That's what the LifestyleChangeWithApril gave to me—a sisterhood with a common goal of creating the best versions of ourselves. In addition to being that virtual voice of encouragement, I learned how to take my eating habits and workout routines to the next level. If you commit to this programme, truly commit to the lifestyle, you will absolutely see results. There is no magic, no tea, no wrap; it is all up to you to decide that you want to change in your life, and put in the work. I'm grateful for the group and programme. Seeing the everyday woman have visible results was a major motivation for me. That alone, let me know that it is possible for me. Seeing real people, not celebrities, who have the same struggles and busy schedules as me, put on a bikini and drop sizes is uplifting! If you're thinking about joining, just do it. You have absolutely nothing to lose and everything to gain and you are worth it! Coach will not give up on you as long as you don't give up on yourself. And even if you do, there is an army of women cheering you on and encouraging and praying for you; so you can't fail.

--Diana

At the beginning of 2016, my prayer to God was for my life to be full of praises to Him more than the year before regardless of any situation I found myself. As I was about to finish, I looked at myself and realised that in order for me to be full of praises to God, I have to be happy within my soul. So, I prayed to reduce my weight and asked God to help me with how to go about it. Fast forward to August 2016, my sister-in-law came into town and she looked really good. She told me about Aprillaugh, how it's not about dieting but lifestyle changes with group of women encouraging each other to achieve their goals. I prayed that God should take total control and I contacted April. She was gracious, humble and very welcoming. I explained my weaknesses, my hereditary diabetes, and she said there's nothing impossible for God. This heavenly group has been another contact I have had with God that keeps confirming He's God. I keep saying to Lola that this group is bigger than her and this is the reason. I have learned so much about patience, humility, women empowerment and gained so much knowledge, wisdom and understanding. I can't believe I have lost all this weight and still keep going.

I joined this programme with the desire to be healthy, but I have sisters with so much love and have made amazing friends. Lola, I appreciate you and your work, humility and your love for God is beyond words. I can't believe I am training for marathon next year, and it's all down to God and April Laugh.

--Morenike A

Morenike A

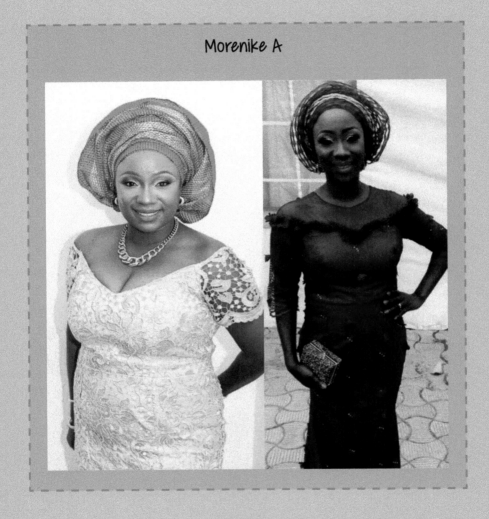

My name is Jare, mom of 3 and on the #LifeStyleChangeWithApril. I came across @fitmrsfats on Instagram when I was just about nine weeks pregnant with my third child. I am your regular overweight mum, always looking for one fad diet or the other, losing weight and then gaining it all back again. It was a cycle I was tired of. With my two previous pregnancies, I had preeclampsia, I will tell you about it shortly. So when I found out I was pregnant and overweight at the time, I knew I had to take control of my health to avoid complications later in the pregnancy. I don't remember what drew me to Lola but I found myself sending her an email and before I knew it, I had signed up and we got chatting. Preeclampsia is a case of high blood pressure in pregnancy, which if not properly monitored, is accompanied by a high degree of protein in the urine which is usually a sign of a malfunctioning kidney. Sounds scary, doesn't it? One of the major causes of preeclampsia is being overweight. Genes, stress, previous history are other factors. But being overweight before conception and into pregnancy is a major factor. This condition can lead to the death of both mother and child before or during delivery, if not properly handled. It is also a major cause of low birth weight and premature births. What it does is this— when the blood pressure is constantly high, the baby stops receiving nutrients from the mother after about 25weeks of pregnancy. In most cases, delivery is usually through surgery and pregnancy which is not carried to full term. This is always the safest option for both lives.

I was lucky to have a good gynaecologist, who noticed early enough with my first 2 pregnancies and handled it well. I was 115kg at 9weeks, my heaviest weight ever and knew I had to do something. My goal was not to add any weight at all through the pregnancy. It sounded impossible to me but I was determined. I don't know what went through Lola's mind when I told her, I even remember saying I wanted to lose weight. She probably didn't see the possibility too. But being the goal getter that she is, she said, just follow my plan and forget about the scale. Focus on eating healthy and being active till the end. And so the journey began, she sent my meal plan, I thought kile leyi (what is this?). Then I saw the exercise routine. I laughed in Swahili.

But I started, because like I said, I was determined. I needed to be healthy enough to handle two toddlers, with a third child on the way. Every day, the exercises got better; I enjoyed the meals too. Difficult at first with portion control and substitutes for things like rice and bread (oh how I love bread!). But seeing results changed everything. I was burning calories like it was nothing. I felt lighter, I felt stronger, and my bump was growing. Best of all, I was losing weight, the scale was shifting. I went from 115KG at 9weeks to 109KG at 36weeks. My doctor was happy, my baby was healthy, my BP was under control. The lifestyle change helped me a lot because I did not stop. Even when I stopped working out at about 32weeks, I still continued to eat healthy. I wish I knew about her before I got pregnant, I would have been at my healthy weight before conception. There's no quick fix, just determination and focus. The support group is beyond amazing, the most down-to-earth people ever. We have the days we struggle, some of us want coke, some want cake, and some want ayamase rice and stew. But when you see abs and weight loss pictures of other group members, you forget those cravings. It won't happen in 7days, give it time and just focus. As I type, it is two weeks post-delivery and I'm waiting for my doctor to give me an all clear to start working out again. I'm breastfeeding presently, and still using her meal plan. Forget all those lies about drinking thick milo and milk to breastfeed. Get her meal plan to fuel your body right, and it will thank you for it. Your body is not a dustbin for junk! You don't need to starve; you can even eat up to five times a day. Looking forward to my December body, I plan to give it my all, the journey has just begun. I have about 45kg to shed to get to my healthy weight, but one day at a time. If I could lose weight while pregnant, how much more now. Take control of your life today with April, you'd be happier for it!

--Jare

I'm a 12-weeker and I just wanted to share a few words about these past 3 months. I know the scale doesn't always sing for us. I'm not thrilled at 8kg loss because I wanted more, but I know I still battle with food but I am so thankful for how my life has changed. My inches loss is amazing, but the health benefits are tenfold. I'm a former pneumonia patient and every month without fail, I would always have a cough and/or cold. I haven't been sick these past 12 weeks or needed my inhaler. My periods are not as viscous as before, and I haven't needed to take sick leave which used to be or rather, was the case. This last change will make you laugh; I had lost my hair through PCOS and medication. I had an honest-to-God bald spot; now, my hair is growing back at a ridiculous rate. I've never seen anything like it. So, I'm here eyeing up the clothes I'm sending to charity shops because they are too big, I want to encourage anyone who may be feeling down. Don't stop the good thing we have started here. The benefits are not just the 'after pictures', the good things are happening on a cellular level too.

--Chizoba

I have never really had a sweet tooth; thank God!! In 2010, I lost 20kg on the Atkins ... It felt good whilst it lasted but I certainly couldn't stay away from carbs, so the weight crept up. Fast forward March 2017, I just felt low and unhealthy; nothing fitted and I got tired so easily... a couple of friends told me about April Laugh and I decided to give it a try... within weeks, I was hooked. I could have breakfast, lunch, dinner and snacks without feeling guilty and it was balanced. I sleep better; my lab results, which once showed a high cholesterol level, is now normal. I look and feel good. My journey isn't over but I am certainly not where I started. I can't sing your praises enough...you have proven that distance is certainly not a barrier to achieve your goals. I am in Ghana, you are in London, but you are always there to lead the way.

Afua

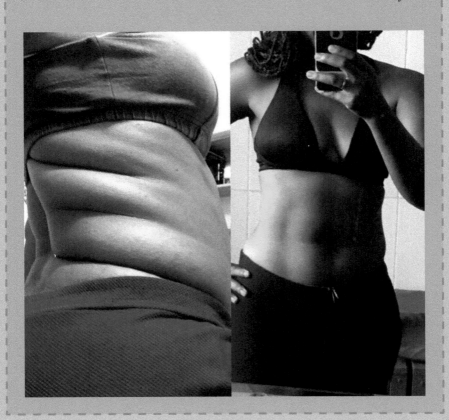

"*Trying to control my weight had been a struggle for as long as I can remember. I was a "well fed baby," you see that toddler who always has an extra bottle of milk... that was me. When we were in uni, being a size 16, I vividly remember arguing with Yello that I couldn't get any bigger; she laughed and told me she'd remind me when I got bigger. Sadly, she got her chance. I've tried quite a number of diets (including the very low calorie diets with soups and shakes), I'd lose some kg but they always seemed to go find more friends and settle right back in, so I almost gave up. Early this year, at a nice, round size 22, I decided to give weight loss one more try and if it didn't work, well, I figured that meant God wanted me to remain well fed. As luck would have it, around that time my sister, introduced me to April but I must confess, I didn't think it would work especially when we calculated my BMI and I needed to lose 36 kg (like that's a whole person). In my mind, I was like... never going to happen but then, I thought... let me just try. Honestly, that was the best and healthiest decision I've ever made. First thing I learnt was that it's not about just weight loss, but a lifestyle change; that way, I'd be able to lose the weight steadily and most importantly, keep the weight off after getting to my ideal weight. Initially, it wasn't easy; in fact, many times, I asked myself... who send you work but with the support of the Coach and amazing April Laugh's sisters (Shout out fab fitfam) I've been able to take it one day at a time and now, I'm over 30kg down... Yay.*

I'm not where I want to be but now, I know it's very possible. I just need to stick to my lifestyle change journey, and I'll get there. Thanks April for helping me turn my life around."

--Tomike

Tomike

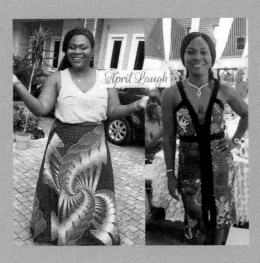

"My name is Lillian, I'm a mum of 3. I met April on Instagram as I was just scrolling up and down. I saw her transformation pic of when she just had her son and her seven months later pic, and I was immediately inspired. I said to myself if she can do this I definitely can because her tommy looked exactly like mine after child birth. (drools) and I was actually pregnant at the time... almost due, so I contacted April and 6 weeks after I had my baby, we started and ever since, it's been amazing. Seeing my body transform in the most amazing ways. That's not to say we perform magic at the LifestyleChangeWithApril. No! We don't. It takes hard work and dedication but it's definitely worth every penny, every tear, every pain, and every sweat I promise you. The meals are also amazing; you still get to eat everything with just few changes here and there. My hubby always beefs me; when I'm prepping my food, he stands there eyeing my big big chicken; Lol. I started seeing changes after 4weeks, and haven't stopped seeing changes in my body. I definitely feel brand new, and loving every single bit of it. Thank you so much Lola; you are one hell of a lady, you are my bad ass, and I love you; and to the amazing ladies on the group, you guys are wonderful. Anyone that goes through LifestyleChangeWithApril and doesn't see changes, definitely hasn't put in work full stop."

--Lillian O

Lillian O

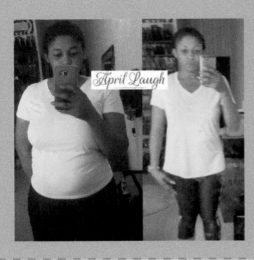

Wow! Where do we start from? As newbies, the veterans welcomed us to the family in Week. 1 don't know what the future holds for us. We came in and we were our own motivators, and a bond was formed; our highs were each other's high as well as our low moments. From weigh-in days to days where the body was not willing to work out. We became the 1k gang to BEASTMODE to #TEAMJUSTDOTHEDAMNTHING. Then we grew into five heads and three heads; WOW! We became family, from sisters to mentors to AL FitHives, we all crushed FAT together as the AM and PM crew. The motivators that kept us on our toes were Nonye, Zita and Tosin, the five head gang. We turned rest days into beastmode days when we heard the pings on our phones.

By week 12, we have grown both physically and spiritually. We have become healthier and stronger. At this point, we would like to say thank you to our teachers, the ones we met in the family, and the ones that have come after us; you make it all complete. We learn from you each day.

To our coach of life, Lola April—you see why we are special? We came in April—thank you for being a selfless, resilient, therapist/motivator. You make it all complete; you make everyone feel special in their own way. You bring out the best in us. We can only say, THANK YOU! The Lord has just started with you.

Finally, to the class of April 2017, I want to wish everyone the best of luck in this healthy journey. For those of us strong enough to go on this healthy journey alone, remember, do not forget us and the support group we have on Facebook. We will miss you. To those of us continuing this journey to the master's level, let us do this! God bless us all!

Love,
OshB for Baddest"

Oshioneh

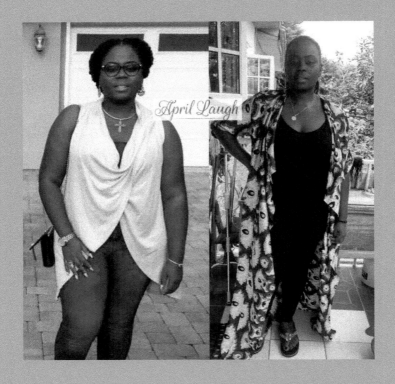

I am speechless right now because I can't really find the exact words to thank all of you for being my inspiration number 1, and for pushing me all the way to show up everyday, even with a 500 – calories burn. You've never teased me; you all have always loved me. I really feel loved; being the youngest in the group and living away from my home, I felt like your love was similar to my mom's. That's why I always showed up too. Thank you so much for everything; it was more than a pleasure to meet y'all. I hope to meet everyone one day in person. Coach, YOU ROCK!! HAIL TO THE QUEEN LOLA. You deserve it. Bringing all of these beautiful and strong women together, and making sure that each one brings out the best in them is a blessing. I pray that God bless abundantly your house, and that he restores everything broken in your life. May He, the Almighty, give His peace to you, the one that goes beyond our understanding. Thank you for bringing out the best in each one of us. I learned so many things here, and surely, I am just starting! I will keep going and make you proud!! Thanks ♥

I will miss everybody. Love you lots ♥

Ester

One of the things that first struck me when we started this journey was April's amazing way of knowing exactly what to say to each one of us just at the right time. You'd post your workout for the day, and she'd follow through with a comment that made you know she was watching and paying attention to every detail. Her words of motivation—along with that of everyone in this group, and of course, all the amazing burns—pushed me to do more. I knew she would be here, checking to make sure I had put in some work for the day. I especially enjoyed her smileys. It always made me laugh. Thanks to her fitness plan; I became more conscious of what I put in my body. When I did not have my food scale yet, I used to go online and check the calories of every single ingredient I put in my food, just to make sure I wasn't overdoing anything. I became more accountable to myself for my weight. Instead of being deeply sad that I wasn't how I used to be, I took strength from the fact that I was working my way up to how I wanted to be. The walks, runs, the exercise routines all revealed to me an inner strength and discipline to stick to a set goal in the long term. It was good to discover this. As days grew into weeks, my self-confidence grew as my shorts fell off my waist. I had never been happier and PROUDER to pull the strings in my shorts tighter around my waist. I was smiling EVERYWHERE I went. I am naturally very self-conscious but now, when I run on the street, I don't care who is looking, because I knew I looked good doing it. I never knew I would enjoy sweating till I begun exercising. The sweat served as proof of all my efforts. I am grateful for all the amazing people I met here: smiling Ester (I still don't know how she managed to smile so sweetly after a serious workout); our motivational PTOSIN, Afua Nkrumah, Nana Konadu and all the lovely ladies with their amazing burns; Chi with her very funny and unique choice of words that was sure to make you laugh always; GS, who tirelessly recorded our figures and was sometimes stern, but always ready with motivation, and Adesholzy, who freely gave us trophies to push us to do more. I am grateful to have been part of this. It helped me on the road to further self-discovery. I lost more than calories, and gained more than a slimmer figure, and for that, I am truly grateful. God bless you, coach, and give you more years to help many more people. And if I ever need help, I will not hesitate to come right back. After all, this is a family in its own right, where all are welcome with open arms. It's been great getting to know you all.

--Barbara

I moved back to UK from US in December 2014, and I had a natural change in schedule. Fast forward to 2016, I decided to shed some weight and get ready for some hot 40 pics. Alas, I could not. I found out I just could not exercise or get in shape. I was very discouraged.

Around January, I saw @GS posting some runs on Instagram, and I kept seeing April's hashtag, so I started following her. I later reached out, spoke to her, she was very personable, so I started with a detox thinking, I would start February but didn't start till March. I can only say I appreciate this lady. I appreciate this group. I have never been a "disciplined eater" because my eating times vary so much. This journey has helped me create more structure and most importantly, motivated me to move constantly. I was excited to see the name of our new group. It's a new challenge. I enjoyed the banter here so much but we will start our own over there.

Thank you ladies for keeping it real. It's been fun. Thank you @ Adesola LWA @GS @Tosin LWA for being awesome support systems for the group. Thank you @Mrs Fats, for obeying the call. You have created 2 platforms, for our physical care and the other for our soul and spirit. May your gift continually make room for you and bring you before kings.

--Adenyke

Wow. I can't believe my transformation myself. Been wanting to lose weight over the last three years but found it very difficult. I will eat right and exercise for a week and the following week, zero. I came across April Laugh around March 2017, and started following her page on Instagram but thought to myself, I bet this is all fake!! (All these Photoshop people). I had my doubts but kept following. However, around May, she did a live video which I happened to view live. The 1st thing I thought was oh! So, she is real. People asked questions and so did I, and I was impressed by the response she gave. As soon as the video ended, I emailed her straight away, and I got a response immediately. However, she was fully booked until July but I kept looking at all the transformation pictures she posted and thought to myself, July can't come any sooner for me. I was so eager to start. So came 1st of July, and I started on this amazing journey. April is the most beautiful person inside and out. The amazing ladies on the group are totally out of this world. The support you get on this journey is absolutely phenomenal. We eat proper and great food, and still lose weight. I remember my son saying "mum, you are not going to lose weight with all this food" but I said to him, watch me shrink. LOL. So far, this journey has been amazing and it's exactly what I needed to be accountable. Just look at these pictures. Wow. I am amazed. Thank you coach; you are one in a million.

--Morenike O

2016, I decided that I was going to do something about my weight instead of calling myself OROBO all the time. I was so used to calling myself OROBO, just so people know that I'm aware of my weight, and they didn't need to remind me about it talk about coping mechanism (Naijas and their "You've added oh!"

The search began for a weight loss coach because I knew I needed someone to be accountable to. I contacted a few, and they made me feel like I was part of a building project I lost hope mehn, and I decided to just embrace my fat self, after all, He prepares a table before me and I didn't want to disobey God by not eating the varieties that he had blessed me with.

One glorious day, I came across @fitmrsfats, who is now my Big Sister I called her on the 2nd of Nov 2016, and she responded sharp sharp I was like ahhh (I was praying she wouldn't so that I'll convince myself that I tried. I'm sure God wasn't having that, and was looking at me like)...

When @fitmrsfats spoke to me, I was like "Osheyy I'll lose weight" until she started telling me things I had to let go.

My apartment was stocked with amazing nonsense. I was heartbroken. I remember being quiet on the phone for like two minutes, and she had to ask if I'm serious about it and willing to do all of that. I was actually having chocolate and chilled coke at the time. We ended the convo with me telling her that I'll start on the 15th Nov 2016 (I had to enjoy all those things before saying goodbye biko. I didn't want to be a Yoruba demon with sudden heartbreak to good food jor) and then, she asked me to send my weight and all to her.

FAM, I thought I was like eighty something until I climbed the scale and saw 95.1kg. I felt like an elephant and then, it occurred to me that I've been rolling all these while (in my head, I've been walking ehh).

The first three weeks were very hard for me, and at the time, we had a WhatsApp group to motivate each other and check progress. She had this thing that puts the fear of God in you. The women on the group are AMAZING!!! These are mothers doing amazing jobs to be fit, and me, I was complaining. No one told me to be serious, from burning 350 cal a day to burning over 1000cal. As the days went by, I felt good, and I started getting compliments, even though I couldn't see nothing in the first four weeks. My clothes got bigger, and I stopped looking like a parachute . I look back at my pictures and I start to laugh (Those of you that said "Damn, hot Mama" God has sha exposed you ohh. I was there looking like Rolling dollar aka Parachute, and you were busy praising me.)

FROM LOOKING LIKE PUFF-PUFF WITH EXCESS YEAST TO ALUMINIUM PLATE OF SMALL CHOPS

--Yetunde

Yetunde

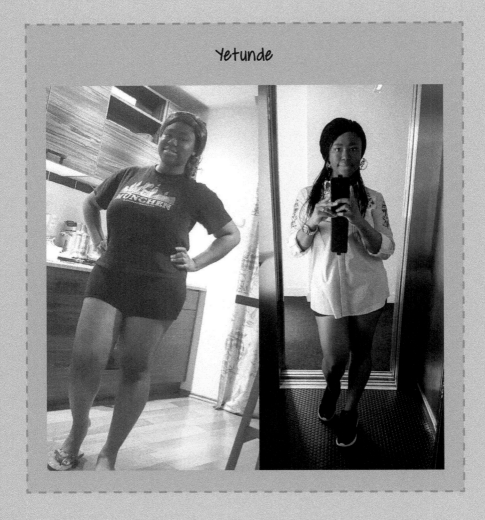

"Before I started following @FitMrsFats on IG, I wasn't sure if it will be a right place for me to start my healthy lifestyle. Compared to a lot of people I saw on her IG page, I was nowhere near them in size, but I knew that something needed to change for me. I was definitely not happy with not only what I looked like, but how I feel about my body.

The idea of working out and eating consistently healthy have always been good, but I thought, how on earth would I have time to go to the gym? And having a wonderful husband that enjoys eating out? When I was approaching 30, we were praying for a different lifestyle. A lifestyle that would allow us to spend more time together as a family, and draw us closer to our heavenly father. So, while I was waiting for this to happen, I thought, why don't I keep myself busy with getting fit and all? So I thought, why not?

I dropped April an email around 10pm just to convince myself if or not I can do this...

April got back to me around 11am next day... I had to wait 12 hrs for her reply...

So, I started; emptied my cupboard and fridge and went for a BIG food shopping... 'chai, healthy food was so expensive,' I thought. Hubby said just do it and stop moaning.

So, what did I learn from this journey 20kg down?

I learnt to cook better

I learnt to dress sexier

I learnt to have self-control, be balanced and self-disciplined.

I feel great

I enjoy exercising

I learnt to motivate others without making them feel uncomfortable.

Now, I'm awake before my alarm goes off at 5am to workout... I can't believe myself that despite my love for sleep, I now wake up early to just get on with the day. Now, two beautiful things are happening in the life of the fit girl.

I can only thank God and April's push to be where I am today, and hoping to continue until God kingdom comes."

--Lillian A

Lillian A

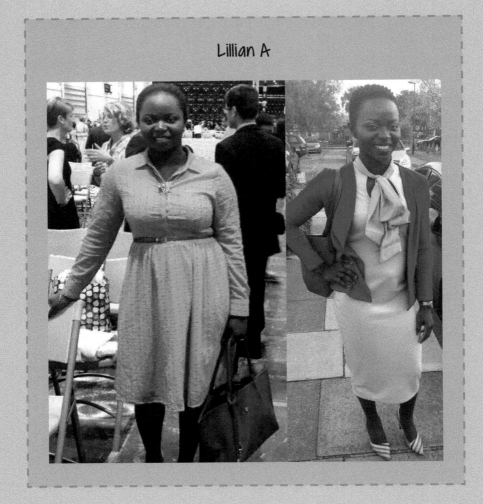

My AL Fitness journey has been one of the most rewarding journeys I've been on. I had been trying (unsuccessfully) for a while to incorporate exercise into my busy lifestyle, but my story changed when I met April.

Beyond getting healthier, fitter and stronger, I have also become a morning person (I nefer hexperredit!), a more disciplined person, and I have also gotten better at time management. Most importantly, I've built some amazing friendships/sisterships with both April, and other members of the AL FitHive. I am still on my journey and I am enjoying it. Some days are hard sha, but we are here for both the 'after' picture and for the personal development.

I love my April and I love my AL FitHive!

--Kemi On

I've always been fat…for as long as I can remember. I can't remember even ever wearing a size 12. I was always easily the biggest in any group, and at some point in my life, I was wearing a size 20/22. I couldn't even do something as easy as crossing my legs, and I used to watch my skinny sister cross hers easily.

And then, I met you April. Bang! My orientation and entire mind-set changed. My lifestyle changed! If anyone told me I could do 3 to 5000 skips, I'd have laughed in their face. If anyone had said I could ever run almost 10km, I'd have asked if they were high. I met you and you've pushed me to do all these and more. I still have a long way to go, but I'm closer to the end than the beginning by God's grace. Trust me, I used to do zero exercise before meeting you, so if I can do this, you can too! April, my heart prays for you. God bless you so much. And thanks to all who have helped and still helping me on this journey

PS: Now I can do centre parting and not be afraid that I'll look like a muppet baby with a fat face.

--Kemi Om

My lifestyle change or fitness journey so far, has been fun, rewarding and a life changing experience.' After having two wonderful girls, it became a struggle to lose weight and to eat three square meals a day. I fell into the habit of eating once a day, and snacking until late. I thought this would help towards my weight loss goals. However, little did I know that I wasn't losing any weight. It was a standstill for me until the Holy Spirit directed me to April. I had already contacted some fitness gurus. But my mind sat on April fitmrsfat, lol. I have not only lost some weight, I have also met some amazing women. Still on my journey until I reach my goal and I am loving it. God bless you richly for changing my life. Yes, you will have some down days. However, consistency is the Golden key.

Esther

Chapter 14

Smash Your Fitness Goals

The days in the new year are runing quickly; where are they even running to? I mean, it feels like it was only last week when we were wishing each other a Happy New Year and praying that we achieve all our goals and plans. How is that going for you? Great, I hope!

For some of you, setting and achieving goals is like a piece of cake or banana bread (healthy options only, please!) while for some of us, it is like trying to break a cement block with our bare hands or ascending Kilimanjaro – tough, challenging, difficult but doable. Physical fitness goals, in particular, are especially more challenging to meet and a lot of us give up after one week – 'we cannot come and go and die, right?' ☺ But it does not have to be a 'dying' affair, at least not for us – the only thing that should be dying is fat.

We have many reasons for giving up on our physical fitness goals but not this year – not anymore. Why, you might ask? What is different about this year? I know the Pastor said it was a year of "insert any prophecy of your

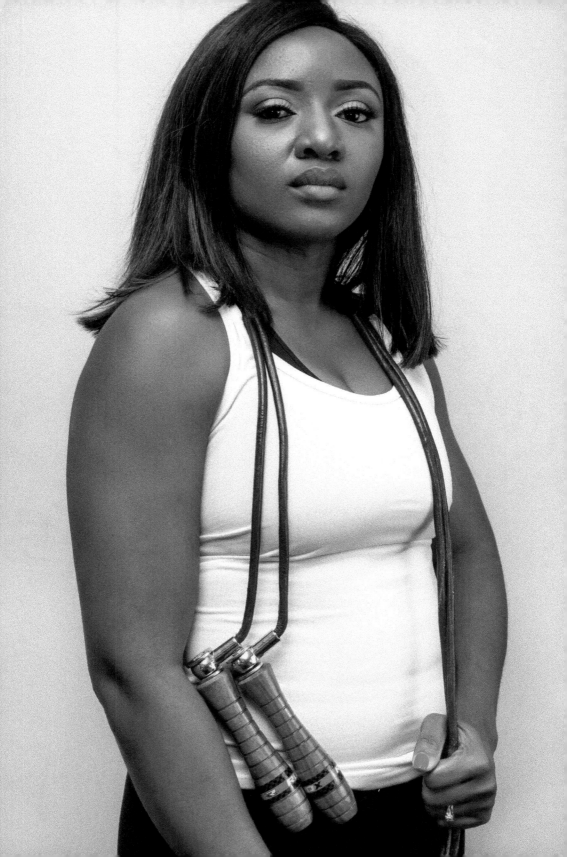

choice here' but that's not the only reason why you are going to meet your physical fitness goals this year. You are going to meet, smash and exceed your goals and you're getting your abs this year because April is here for you. Can I get an Amen?

Lifestyle Change with April keeps it simple for you; we do all the hardwork for you well, except cooking your meals and working out on your behalf but trust us, if we could, we would. We have the catalogue of all the possible excuses you might give and we have the answers for all of them.

- *Oh April, I have a very busy schedule.* #Wehdone Ma, #Wehdone Sir, we have some of the busiest bankers, lawyers, doctors, consultants and entrepreneurs on our team making time to prepare meals on weekends and ensuring they exercise every day, even at the oddest hours. Oyebola is a banker, we did that in 12 weeks!
- *Oh April, there is no gym in my area.* Clap for yourself. After clapping, send us an email. Once you sign up, we will tailor your exercise regime around your lifestyle. You might never have to visit a gym before you meet your abs. Trust us! Lillian is a new mom and we did that without stepping in the gym.
- *Oh April, I live in the Antarctica and won't be able to meet you personally for coaching.* Don't worry. We have clients located all around the world – HongKong, Australia, the U.S, Nigeria, Ghana, Cameroon – and we are working with all of them as they push to achieve their goals. *singing* Distance is no barrier, come and join us. Yetunde lives in Hungary and we achieved that in 8 weeks!
- *Oh April, I have weak knees and can't run.* Sorry to break your heart hun, but we got something special for you too. Slide into our mailbox and we will tell you how we can make it work for you. Genevieve is a new mom and we achieved that in less than 12 weeks!
- *Oh April, without a personal trainer, I can't be great.* Ah, we guess

you haven't heard about us. We are monitoring spirits, working very closely with you to make sure you don't slack off. Plus, you have the advantage of having multiple personal trainers keeping you accountable every step of the way. Tomike sacked her personal trainer the week she joined. She lost 30kg in 9 months!

- *Oh April, I don't like all these fitfam foods – they are too bland.* Wait till you see the delicious meal plan and recipes we offer. You will come back to testify.
- *Oh April, I am a guy and can't be caught dead doing all these girly exercises.* We got you bro. FitMrFats is 100% hunk and he is waiting for you.

Okay, we think you get the point now. You have NO excuses not to achieve your physical fitness goals this year.

The Lifestyle Change with April offers:

- One on one initial consultation to determine your current activity levels and lifestyle
- A practical and effective weight loss plan tailored specially for and specifically to you
- Workout regime guidance to complement your lifestyle and achieve your health goals
- Accountability from day 1 till your goals are achieved
- Constant support and advice all through the 12-week period to help keep you on track and motivated
- Fortnight progress reviews
- Speedy response to queries or questions.

Regardless of who you are—yummy mummy trying to get her groove back, the Oga Boss who wants to become a hunk, the bachelorette trying to fit into a wedding dress, the fine girl who now wants to be a fit sexy girl, the couple who wants to keep fit and maintain a healthy lifestyle together, people on doctor's orders to lose weight—and what level of fitness you currently are at, the Lifestyle Change with April team will work with you to ensure you achieve those fitness goals. Remember, the goal is not being skinny; the goal is to be fit and healthy enough to enjoy life and achieve all your other goals.

Warning: This is not a fad diet or MMM for weight-loss – this is a lifestyle change.

We look forward to meeting you and helping you achieve your goals. How can you find us to sign up?

Email: info@aprillaugh.co.uk
Website: http://aprillaugh.co.uk
Instagram: http://www.instagram.com/fitmrsfats

References

1. NHS: http://www.nhs.uk/Conditions/Binge-eating/Pages/Introduction.aspx
2. Diet Plan for Weight Loss: http://www.dietplanforweightlosscoach.com/5-holiday-weight-loss-tips/
3. American Journal of Clinical Nutrition: http://www.shape.com/weight-loss/tips-plans/holiday-weight-loss-tips
4. Anne Lamott: https://www.goodreads.com/quotes/6830146-almost-everything-will-work-again-if-you-unplug-it-for

April

Detox Guide

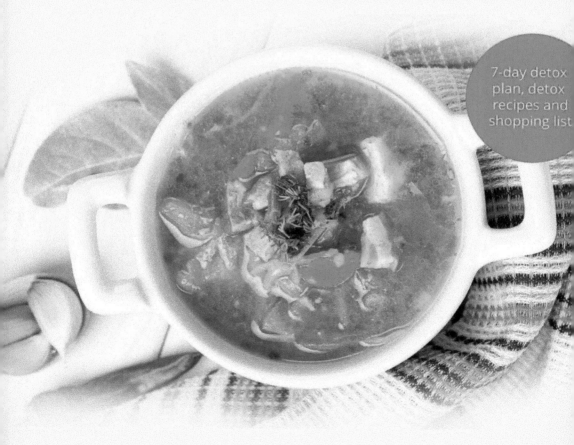

7-day detox plan, detox recipes and shopping list

Table of Contents

Introduction   175
Why Detox?   177
Daily Schedule   181
Frequently Used Recipes   183
Detox Plan   187
List of Ingredients   189
Smash Your Fitness Goals   190

Introduction

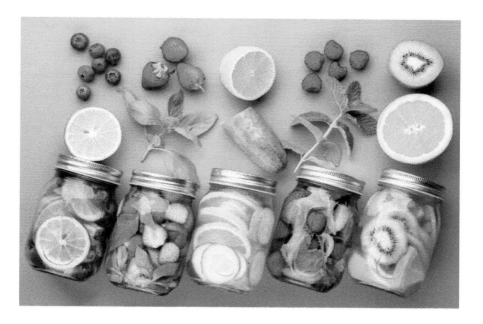

Before I introduce you to this detox plan, you have to prep yourself mentally and physically, this is very important to the success of this plan. A few days before you plan to start, you should make sure you have done the following:

1. Convince yourself you are doing it for the right reasons and be determined on what you intend to achieve
2. Drink 8-10 glasses of water each day to prime the body to shed weight as well as perform detox activities
3. Stock up on foods you need for the next 7 days
4. And lastly, READ THROUGH THE GUIDELINES BELOW:

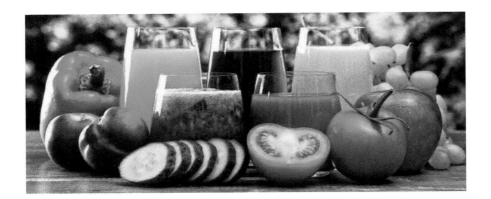

Why Detox?

- Make your eyes sparkle
- Make your skin glow
- Cleanse Your Way Into a healthier Lifestyle
- Boost energy levels
- Improve your digestion
- Shed a few unwanted pounds.

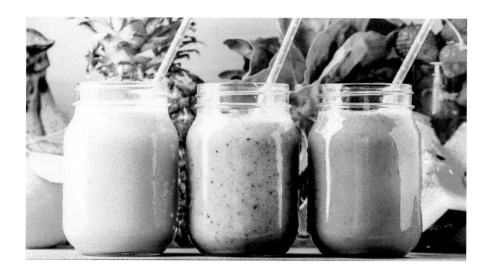

Please note that going on a detox is far from a quick fix for weight loss. The purpose of this detox plan is to detoxify your body while taking some load off your organs – the liver, kidneys and bowel – while at the same time supporting and improving their performance. If you want to fast track your health, give your body a break, or just want to detox diet for a short time, follow this safe and do-able seven-day program. I do this every year or after a holiday and always lose over 5lbs in 3 days. All the people that have bought and participated in this detox have also lost amazing weight in such a short time.

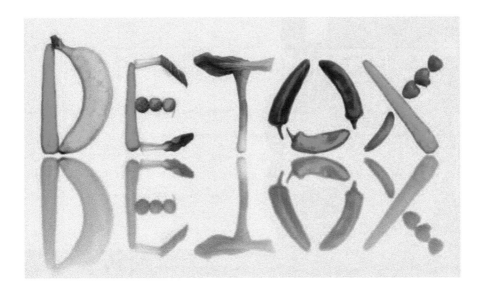

IMPORTANT - EXERCISE Guide:

Besides drinking loads of water during this detox, exercising is also as crucial. Exercise is an important part of any detoxification programme. Move your body to breathe, stretch, circulate and sweat, so the skin can sweat and the kidneys can effectively filter toxins. By increasing your water intake, as well as increasing your heart and breathing rate, your body can more effectively flush out unwanted toxins, fat and waste.

Types of Exercise for Detox: You need a low- intensity aerobic exercise like running, walking, cycling, dancing and swimming. However, you need to go at a pace that helps you breathe evenly and carry on a conversation. Yoga poses are also beneficial because some are specific for detoxifying certain organs. For effective results, pick a form of exercise that you know you will be able to enjoy and start slowly. Exercise for at least 30 minutes five times during the week so your weight can be maintained successfully.

IMPORTANT - Personal Note

This detox plan is high fiber with all the fruits and vegetables in it, you should drink at least 8 glasses of water throughout the day. This would help with emptying your bowel every morning, if this is not the case drink lots more water and Green tea or Twining's Lemon & Ginger: This revitalizing tea is great for the morning because it has light caffeine levels; it will wake you up without wreaking havoc on your stomach. It also limits your cravings later.

IMPORTANT - Medical Notice

If you suffer from any health condition, please talk to your Doctor before embarking on any detox plan. Don't detox if you are pregnant, elderly, suffer from high blood pressure, suffer from diabetes, are underweight or have been advised against detox by your Doctor

IMPORTANT - Legal Notice

DAILY SCHEDULE

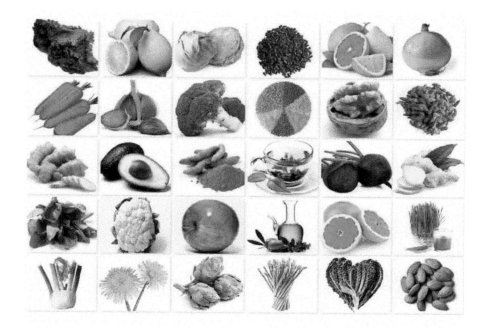

This detox plan is restrictive unlike the meal plans on the LifestyleChangeWithApril. You're allowed to enjoy the following daily:

- Detox Drink
- Water
- Fruits
- Green tea/Twinning's Lemon & Ginger Tea

Daily To DOS

Morning Detox Drink: Take a glass of mild warm water and add 2 teaspoons of Honey and 3 Tablespoons of freshly squeezed lemon juice, mix it well and drink it before breakfast once daily for all 7 days.

Throughout the Day: Drink water. Add your favourite fruits in your water to keep it interesting.

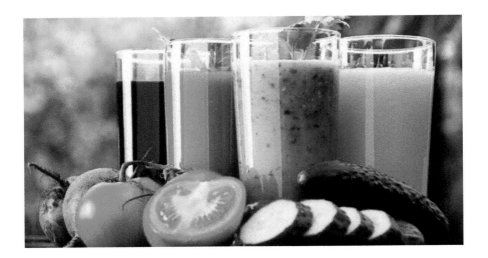

FREQUENTLY USED RECIPES

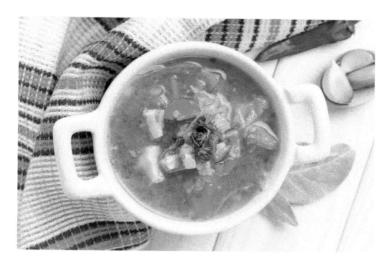

Detox Drink

Take a glass of mild warm water and add 2 teaspoons of Honey and 3 Tablespoons of freshly squeezed lemon juice, mix it well and drink.

April's Cabbage Soup

*Serves 4 – 220 Calories Per Serving & SO AMAZING!!!!!

Ingredients: Cabbage- 1 Head
Bell Peppers- 2 Pieces
Tomatoes- 3 Large
Onions- 3 Large
Chicken Broth- 1 1/2cup
Sunflower Oil - 2 Tbsps
Water - 2 cups
Celery - 5 Sticks Season as desired.

Cooking Guidelines:

1. Chop all ingredients finely separately
2. Fry onions with oil, add celery, bell peppers, and tomatoes for few minutes.
3. Add chicken broth, maggie and pepper soup seasonings or any of your choice.
4. Simmer for 2 minutes
5. Add the cabbage, and water.
6. Cook for 30 minutes and serve.

OTHER RECIPES:

Foods to enjoy during the Detox

Fruits: Fruits! Fruits! Fruits! You must know by now that fruits are very important for your health. On this detox, this will improve the healing process and help with an achievable healthy weight loss. Grapefruit is the best weight loss fruit. It has low sugar content and lots of fiber to help improve your digestive system.

Apple: Always try to eat fresh and wax-free apples. Apple alone is not very helpful in healthy weight loss but combined with other fruits, it forms an essential part of healthy fruit diet.

Vegetables: Any and all fresh vegetables

Fish, Turkey, Chicken (without the skin). Limit to two serves for the week.

Smoothies

Morning Fix:
2 cups of spinach
2 cups of Almond milk
2 cups of frozen pineapple
1 Banana

Citrus Breeze
2 cups of spinach
1 1/2 cups of water
2 Oranges
Half mango
1/2 cup of Pineapples
1 Banana

Almond Goodness
2 cups of fresh spinach
2 cups of almond milk
1 banana
Tsp Cinnamon
Berries or Cherries

Clean Juices

Force Field

Ingredients
Beet Root - 1 beet (2" dia) 82g
Carrots - 6 medium 366g
Coconut Water - 1/2 cup 120g
Ginger Root - 1 thumb (1" dia) 24g

Lime - 1/4 fruit (2" dia) 16.75g
Orange - 1 fruit (2-5/8" dia) 131g
Turmeric Root - 2 thumb (1" dia) 48g
Directions: Process all ingredients in a juicer, shake or stir and serve.

Ginger Love

Ingredients
Apple - 1 medium (3" dia) 182g
Carrots - 4 medium 244g
Ginger Root - 1 thumb (1" dia) 24g
Directions: Process all ingredients in a juicer, shake or stir and serve.

Apple Berry

Ingredients
Apple - 1 medium (3" dia) 182g
Carrots - 7 medium 427g
Strawberry (heaping) - 1 cup, whole 144g
Directions: Process all ingredients in a juicer, shake or stir and serve.

DETOX PLAN

	Pre-Breakfast	Breakfast	Lunch	Dinner
DAY 1	Detox Drink	Fruit Bowl	Fruit Bowl	Fruit Bowl
DAY 2	Detox Drink	Fruit Bowl	Fruit Bowl	Fruit Bowl
DAY 3	Detox Drink	Fruit Bowl	Fruit Bowl	Fruit Bowl
DAY 4	Detox Drink	4 Bananas & a glass of Semi-Skimmed Milk	4 Bananas & a glass of Semi-Skimmed Milk	Cabbage Soup
DAY 5	Detox Drink	Citrus Breeze	Grilled Tomatoes With 100g of Grilled Fish or Meat	Cabbage Soup
DAY 6	Detox Drink	Almond Goodness	Chosen Salad (No Dressing) With 100g of Grilled Fish or Meat	Cabbage Soup
DAY 7	Detox Drink	Any Clean Juice	Chosen Salad (No Dressing) With 100g of Grilled Fish or Meat	Cabbage Soup

FRUITS FOR DAY 1 - 3

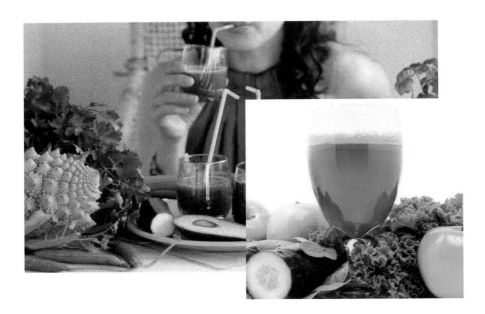

Your typical day should look like:

Early morning (6-9 a.m.) Detox Drink

Breakfast (9 a.m. to 10a.m An unlimited amount of any of the following fruits: Apples, Pineapple, Figs, Pears, Grapes, Kiwi, and Cucumber

Lunch (12 -2p.m.): Oranges or Tangerines, Peaches, and Papayas in any amount desired

Dinner (6p.m.): Mango, Cherries, Strawberries, Red Plums, Watermelon, Grapes, Mango, Persimmons, Pomegranates, and Tomatoes.

NOTE: You are allowed to eat all types of fruits from day 1-3 except Bananas. Whenever you're hungry, you can eat any of the aforementioned fruits.

INGREDIENTS LIST

INGREDIENT	QUANTITY	NOTE
Apples	6	
Pineapples	2	
Kiwis	6	
Tangerines	10	
Mangoes	6	
Pomegranate	3	
Grapefruit	3	
Papayas	2	
Strawberries	1 Bowl	
Bananas	8	
Cabbage	1 head	
Bell Peppers	2	
Tomatoes	6	
Onions	3	
Sunflower Oil		
Celery Sticks	4	
Honey		
Lemon	8	
Twinnings lemon & Ginger Tea		
Green Tea		
Semi-Skimmed Milk		Can be replaced with any plant based milk or natural yogurt.
Fish	200g	
Chicken	200g	
Fresh Salad Greens	As desired	
Spinach	As Desired	
Beetroot	3-5	

Smash your fitness goals

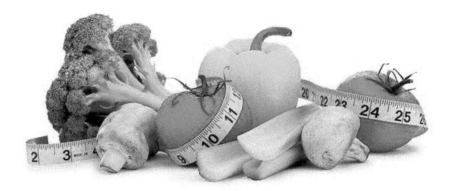

Reflections: Can you believe you made it? You might feel a little weak on the last day because your body has not consumed too much carbohydrate in the last couple of days. Before you go to bed tonight, reflect on the last 7 days and think about your strength and perseverance to stick to this diet. The benefits are tremendous – and affects more than the number you will see on the scale the next morning or the difference in the fit of your clothes. The change will be in the functioning of your body, which will be operating in an enhanced manner due to the detox process.

You can repeat this detox every other month if you choose. Once in two months would be an efficient and healthy way to lose a few pounds that creep up on you when you are not paying attention!

Want More? Sign up for the Lifestyle Change with April.